CONQUERING BACK PAIN

CONQUERING BACK PAIN

Donald Norfolk

BLANDFORD PRESS
POOLE · NEW YORK · SYDNEY

First published in the UK 1986 by Blandford Press,
Link House, West Street, Poole, Dorset, BH15 1LL

Copyright © 1986 United Health Promotion Ltd

Distributed in the United States by
Sterling Publishing Co., Inc.,
2 Park Avenue, New York, NY 10016

Distributed in Australia by
Capricorn Link (Australia) Pty Ltd,
PO Box 665, Lane Cove, NSW 2066

British Library Cataloguing in Publication Data

Norfolk, Donald
    Conquering back pain.
    1. Backache
    I. Title
    616.7'3   RD768

ISBN 0 7137 1740 8

Typeset by Lovell Baines Ltd, Hollington Farm, Woolton Hill,
Newbury, Berkshire.

Printed in Great Britain by Biddles Ltd, Guildford. Surrey.

To my patients who, for thirty years,
have been a never failing source
of encouragement and support;
and to St Laurence,
the patron saint of
back pain sufferers

CONTENTS

1 The Agony Column

Backache is one of man's perennial problems: a malady as widespread as the common cold, as painful as piles and at times as crippling as a stroke. Surveys reveal that four out of every five people around the world will be incapacitated by severe backache at some time in their lives. In the USA the disease has reached epidemic proportions, claiming an estimated 75 million victims, including 2 million whose spinal problems are so severe that they are incapacitated for work. In the UK nearly a third of people suffer an episode of backache in any given fortnight. Most take some form of self-help treatment, but only one or two in every fifty bother to consult their doctors. The treatments they take are notable mainly for their variety and eccentricity. Some wear copper bangles, others carry a slice of potato in their pockets or circle their waists with a band of pink ribbon. A British barrister tries to keep his lumbago at bay by filling his socks with sulphur, a remedy which is more likely to deter his clients than to ward off rheumatism. A Yorkshire businessman sits on a tortoise, a remedy he picked up when he was working in Kenya. 'Doctors failed to cure my back', he reported, 'then a Kikuyu, reputed to be a witch-doctor, brought me the tortoise. It worked.'

Some of these old folk cures appear to offer conflicting advice. Many advocate the elimination of rhubarb from the diet because of its high content of oxalic acid. According to one compendium of country cures: 'Under no circumstances should those who suffer from rheumatism drink rhubarb wine as that makes the condition worse'. Yet another ancient remedy – Lord Anson's potion – consists of a hefty dose of rhubarb mixed with honey, sulphur and cream of tartar. Lord Anson was an eighteenth-century British admiral, famous in his day for his circumnavigation of the globe and his defeat of the French at the battle of Cape Finisterre. He derived so much benefit from taking a daily draught of the rhubarb mixture that he bought the secret recipe for £300, a king's ransom in those days, and made it public as his contribution to the well-being of the nation.

Many cures have their roots in ancient witchcraft. In the UK there is an old Cornish remedy that evokes the protective power of the magic circle. Outside the quaintly named village of Lanyon Quoit, there is a doughnut-shaped boulder called the Men-an-Tol. Anyone who wants to overcome their backache is told to crawl through the stone's central hole without making contact with its sides. The original reason for performing this feat was to escape from the painful clutches of the devil, who couldn't pass through a magic circle. A similar remedy exists in Germany, where sufferers from lumbago are encouraged to make a pilgrimage to the church of St Michael in Bamberg, where they perform the ritual of clambering through the tiny gap in the tomb of Bishop Otto of Pommern, who died early in the twelfth century and gave instructions that, when he died, he was to be buried in such a way that he could be easily contacted by sufferers from lumbago. In keeping with his instructions, his sarcophagus was constructed rather like a knee-hole desk. Many sufferers from chronic back pain find relief after clambering through the sacred gap in Otto's tomb.

Other cures for lumbago are more obvious examples of faith healing. Erasmus of Rotterdam, the great Dutch scholar and humanist, suffered a severe back strain in 1514, when his horse shied on a journey from Ghent to Basel. His groom helped him to dismount but he was in so much pain that he was unable to put one foot in front of the other. So he prayed to the Apostle Paul. If St Paul would give him deliverance from his infirmity, he would make recompense by preparing an up-to-date version of the Epistle to the Romans. Within minutes his prayers were answered and he was able to remount his horse. (One suspects that St Paul might have preferred to leave him incapacitated by the roadside had he known in advance how he would maltreat his famous text!)

Doctors today are anxious to adopt a more scientific approach to the treatment of back pain. Before they instigate treatment they always try to establish an accurate diagnosis. This is not easy because there are over a hundred separate causes of back pain, which often overlap and rarely present an unequivocal clinical picture.

Some of the common causes of back pain are:

☆ *Muscle Tension* The lower part of the back is often the site of sustained muscular contraction. As one doctor has said: 'Lumbago is often a tension headache which has slipped lower down the back'.

☆ *Ligament Strain* The postural strain of standing for long periods with the back arched, or of sitting in a slumped position, can provoke ligament strain.

☆ *Spinal Deformity* A lateral deformity of the spine (scoliosis), an excessive rounding of the upper back (kyphosis) or an exaggerated hollowing of the lumbar spine (lordosis) can increase the risk of postural strain but these in themselves are not an inevitable cause of back pain.

Patients often resign themselves to a lifetime of suffering because they have a spinal deformity. This is no more valid than saying that you have to be neurotic because you lost your parents when you were 12 years old, or that you must suffer sunburn in the summer because you have fair skin. Research at the University of Copenhagen has shown that uncomplicated scoliosis is just as common in pain-free subjects as it is in patients suffering from backache.

☆ *Disc Injury* The treatment of back injuries suffered a setback in 1934, when two orthopaedic surgeons disclosed that spinal nerve pain could result from the pressure of a prolapsed disc. (Discs are the fibrocartilaginous shock absorbers interspersed between the vertebrae.) Since that time, there has been a tendency to ascribe all severe back pains and sciaticas to a 'slipped' disc, a blanket diagnosis which is as accurate and as valid as attributing all cases of indigestion to gastric carcinoma. The truth is that disc prolapses are exceedingly common and are more often painless than a source of discomfort.

☆ *Lumbar Spondylosis* With the passage of time, the spine undergoes certain degenerative changes; the discs thin, the spinal joints become arthritic and bony spurs, known as osteophytes, develop around the bodies of the vertebrae. These changes make their appearance in the late 20s and early 30s and are so common in people over the age of 60 years that they might be taken as the norm rather than the exception. All too often, patients with backache are told that they must resign themselves to the situation, because their X-rays show signs of irreversible degenerative change but, in fact, tests show that X-ray evidence of lumbar spondylosis is just as common in pain-free subjects as in patients complaining of low back pain.

☆ *Facet Injuries* In 1927, a paper was published in a medical journal pointing out that back pain could result from injuries to the facet joints on either side of the spine. These tiny joints are easily damaged by torsional strains. When this happens, the joints swell, just like a damaged ankle or knee, and this can cause painful pressure on the emerging spinal nerves.

It would be easy to go on elaborating the numerous mechanical causes of back pain. This might be of interest to some readers, but is of little practical value. This is not a textbook of anatomy, nor is it a manual of orthopaedic pathology. Most family doctors admit that they find it impossible to differentiate between the various causes of lumbago, so what chance has the layman of making an accurate diagnosis? As one Cambridge doctor wrote in a recent issue of the *Practitioner*: 'The doctor will rarely be able to make a diagnosis beyond "non-specific back pain".' Mercifully this is no great drawback. You don't have to understand the intricacies of electronic technology to operate a micro-computer, nor do you have to understand the patho-physiology of the human spine to overcome back pain. All that is necessary is to follow certain tried and tested remedies. These will give relief from back pain and sciatica in the vast majority of cases, without the need for injections, surgery or prolonged courses of hospital treatment.

The first treatise carrying advice for back-pain sufferers was the Edwin Smith Papyrus. This was written nearly 5,000 years ago, possibly by Imhotep, the physician-architect who was responsible for the building of the step-pyramid at Sakkara and who must have treated the strained backs of many of his labourers. When archaeologists pieced together the fragments of this parchment, they decoded the following advice: 'Treatment: you should place him prostrate on his back. You should make him ...'. At that tantalising point the hieroglyphic record ends. This book carries on where the Edwin Smith Papyrus left off! It gives practical advice to patients crippled with a sudden bout of acute back pain, which the Germans appropriately refer to as a *hexenschuss* or 'witch's blow', and carries step-by-step guidance on how to overcome chronic lumbago and sciatica. The message is essentially one of hope. The majority of cases of back pain get better spontaneously, three-quarters within a week. Those which persist, and equally well those which recur, are invariably the product of mishandling rather than mischance. People become chronic sufferers not because they are incurable but because they are not cured. The word chronicity comes from the Latin root *chronos* (meaning time) and refers to the length of time a condition has persisted, rather than to its inevitable resistance to cure.

Because you were crippled with backache yesterday doesn't mean that you are going to be incapacitated for the remainder of your life. Garry Muhrcke was invalided out of the New York Fire Service because of severe back problems. A few years later he had made such an excellent recovery that he was able to enter a gruelling race up the 1,575 steps of the Empire State Building. Competing with fifteen other marathon runners, he was the first to reach the top of the eighty-six-floor skyscraper in the remarkable time of 12 minutes 32 seconds. Not bad for a man who was once incapacitated with lumbago!

There is no need to be a martyr to back pain if you follow the guidance given in this book, which is based on over 30 years' experience in a busy osteopathic practice. But you must genuinely want to be cured. Some people enjoy the sympathy they get when they advertise their aches and pains. Others find back pain a useful excuse for avoiding uncongenial work. Because of their backs they can't garden, lift, iron, wash-up, go to work, make love or travel long distances by car. If you welcome this convenient alibi, you can throw this book away. Overcoming back pain requires a considerable investment in effort and time. The benefit you get from the pages which follow will be directly proportional to the strength of your determination to be cured.

Getting better often means overcoming unconscious mental blocks. Doctors sometimes unwittingly cast a spell over their patients, telling them that they must resign themselves to a lifetime of backache because of their age, their old spinal injuries, their sway-back, their arthritis or their degenerating discs. This is rarely true but can become a self-fulfilling prophecy. At other times people are encouraged to make a virtue of accepting a lifetime of semi-invalidism. 'You'll be fine providing you don't bend, lift weights or walk over uneven ground', some are told. This is tantamount to a garage mechanic saying: 'Your car will be alright providing you don't take it up hills or try to drive it faster than 30 mph'. In the same way it is little consolation to be told 'You won't notice you've got back pain if you continue to take these analgesic pills'. This is no better than telling a motorist, 'Wear these ear muffs and you won't hear your big end knocking'.

The only worthwhile aim is to be fully mobile, totally active and completely free of back pain. This is a realistic goal, if you care passionately enough about the final result and are prepared to observe the instructions which follow.

2 'The Witch's Blow'

All men are born equal but some are born more equal than others when it comes to suffering from back pain. A number come into the world with structural deformities and defects which render them prone to spinal problems. Others are genetically destined to be tall and thin, which makes them particularly liable to postural strain and back injuries. But these inherited tendencies are trivial compared with the predispositions we acquire as we journey through life. Back pain is largely a disorder of life style. At birth we have the spines our parents give us; at 40 years old, we have the spines we deserve. Lumbago has become the endemic disease of the age because we lead uncongenial lives which encourage stiff joints, flabby muscles, postural strain, tension and obesity.

Bouts of backache do not appear without reason. There is no mystery about them. They are not sent by the gods as punishments for misdeeds, as our forebears believed. They are due to straightforward mechanical causes and, as such, are both predictable and explicable.

You can get a good indication of your liability to backache by completing the following test, devised especially for this book.

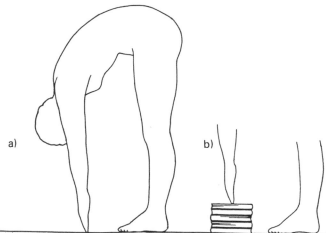

Figure 1 Flexibility test: a) reaching to the ground with knees straight b) measuring the gap between the fingertips and toes.

14

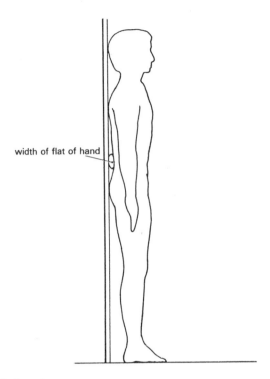

width of flat of hand

Figure 2 Ideal standing posture.

Back Pain Risk Assessment Test

Subject	Question	Points scored for 'yes' answer
Occupation	Does your work involve repeated bending, twisting, heavy lifting or load carrying?	2
Weight	Are you more than 1 stone (6.4kg) overweight? Are you more than 2 stone (12.7kg) overweight? (Score for only one of these questions)	1 2
Flexibility	Stand with knees straight and reach down to touch your toes (see Figure 1a). If you cannot reach the ground, use a pile of paperback books to measure the gap between your fingers and toes (Figure 1b). Gap less than 2 in (5 cm) Gap 2–4 in (5–10 cm) Gap more than 4 in (10 cm)	1 1½ 2

Subject	Question	Points scored for 'yes' answer
Driving	Do you regularly drive more than 100 miles (160 km) per week?	1
Smoking	Do you smoke? Less than 20 a day? More than 20 a day? (Score for only one of these questions)	½ 1
History	Have you suffered backache in the past? Did you suffer from backache before you were 20 years old? Have you ever been confined to bed because of severe back pain? (Score for each of these questions)	1 1 2
Posture	Stand with your back to wall as shown in the diagram, with your feet 4 in (10 cm) from the skirting board and with your head, shoulder blades and buttocks touching the wall (see Figure 2). In this position is the gap between the wall and the small of your back greater than the thickness of your flat hand?	1
Body build	Are you tall and thin?	1
Abdominal muscles	Lie face upwards on the floor with your feet tucked up under a convenient piece of furniture or held by a friend. Now try to bring yourself up into the sitting position: A. With your hands folded across your chest. B. With hands clasped behind your neck and arms parallel to the ground. Are you able to perform test A? Are you able to perform test B? (Score for only one of these questions) See Figure 3.	2 1

Assessment	Less than 5 points	Low risk
	5–10 points	Medium risk
	Over 10 points	High risk

Whatever your showing on this test, you can improve the health of your back by following the practical advice contained within this book: the higher your score, the more urgent your need to embark upon this programme of rehabilitation.

Since you have shown the interest to buy, borrow or acquire a copy of this book, the chances are that you are already suffering from chronic or recurrent backache. In this case, you can browse through the book at your leisure and discover the prophylactic measures that are most

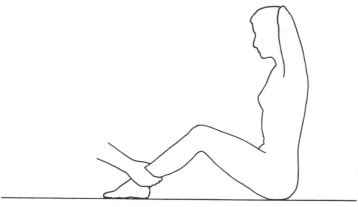

Figure 3 Testing the strength of the abdominal muscles.

appropriate to ease your pains. If you are in a hurry to make progress, you may spotlight your particular problem by answering the following questionnaire.

Does your back hurt when you stand?	
This may mean: a) That your posture is poor.	(see pp.30–34)
b) That you art overweight.	(see pp.19–21)
c) That your tummy muscles are weak.	(see pp.39–44)
Is your pain made worse by sitting?	
This may mean: a) You are sitting in a bad posture.	(see pp.39–44)
b) Your spine is too stiff to flex properly.	(see pp.67–73)
Do you get pain when bending forward weeding the garden, ironing, or preparing food in the kitchen?	
This may mean: a) Your spine is too stiff to flex properly.	(see pp.67–73)
b) Your work surfaces are too low.	(see pp.79)
Are you uncomfortable lying on your stomach? Does it hurt to lie on your back and raise both legs?	
This suggests that your back is too hollow.	(see pp.31–32)
Do you feel better when you have had a hot bath?	
This may mean: a) Your back muscles are stiff.	(see pp.100–103)
b) You are holding yourself with too much tension.	(see pp.81–86)
Did your pain follow a heavy fall or lifting strain?	
This may mean that you suffered an injury which healed imperfectly with stiffness and adhesions.	(see pp.67–73)
Is your back stiff and painful when you get out of bed in the morning, but gets quickly better when you start to move about?	
This may mean: a) You are sleeping on a bad bed.	(see pp.50–53)
b) Your back is insufficiently supple and grows stiffer with the relative immobility of a night's rest.	(see pp.67–73)
Does driving make your back pain worse?	
This may be due to tension, an uncomfortable driving seat or excessive vibration.	(see pp.45–49)
Is your pain made worse by walking over irregular ground or on inclines?	
This suggests that you may have insufficient flexibility in your hip joints.	(see pp.62–66)

If you suffer an acute episode of back pain or sciatica, which gives you severe pain, limits your movements, disturbs your sleep and makes it painful to walk, dress and cough, you will need immediate help. You won't have either the inclination or the time to scan through this book for helpful advice. Here are the emergency measures you should take:

First Aid Relief For Acute Lumbago And Sciatica

Bed rest	Spend 24–48 hours in bed	(see pp.96–99)
Traction	Stretching can sometimes help to relieve the pressure on trapped spinal nerves	(see pp.94)
Support	Comfort can be gained by supporting the back with a belladonna plaster	(see pp.145)
	corset or wide body belt.	(see pp.98–99)
Pain relief	Can be obtained with drugs	(see pp.115–116)
	counter irritation	(see pp.110–112)
	acupressure	(see pp.119)
	cold sprays and packs	(see pp.122–123)
	controlled breathing	(see pp.143)
	mustard packs	(see pp.138)
	autosuggestion	(see pp.144)

With these aids, the majority of episodes of acute back pain should subside within 3–5 days. Those that persist require skilled investigation and treatment from an experienced doctor, osteopath or chiropractor. If any of the following symptoms arise, medical help *must* be sought:

If you experience any disturbance of bowel or bladder functioning.
If you suffer numbness or pins and needles in the region of the anus and genital organs, a site often described as the saddle area.
If you suffer pain which is unrelated to movements and changes of posture.
If you have a rash, high temperature or any other symptom of general ill-health.

Once your acute pain has subsided, you should adopt a prophylactic programme of back care to ensure that you do not suffer a relapse. Never be content to remain a lifetime sufferer from chronic backache or a victim of recurrent attacks of severe lumbago. Never allow your work or social life to be impaired by spinal disorders. Invariably there is a satisfactory answer to these distressing problems. If you don't find it in the pages of this book, as I hope and expect, seek expert advice.

3 A Slim Chance

We are living in a sedentary age in which a large percentage of the population is under-exercised and overweight. Most people put on weight as they grow older, developing a thickened waistline, flabby thighs, pudgy buttocks and double chin. The development of this middle-aged spread would be of purely cosmetic interest were it not for the fact that it predisposes to a wide variety of sicknesses. People who are 10 per cent overweight are more than twice as likely to suffer symptoms of chronic ill health, such as fatigue, shortness of breath, indigestion and back pain.

The grossly obese have no idea of the strain they impose on their spines. It is not uncommon for me to see patients who are 8 stone (50 kg) overweight. Sometimes, their bodies have coped with this burden for years without complaint, but eventually the strain tells and their overloaded backs cry out for help. Corpulent folk like this often come to me expecting a miracle cure but the remedy generally lies less in my hands than in theirs, which they really ought to tie behind their backs every time they sit down to eat! Frequently I ask them to imagine how they would feel if they had to carry a 1 cwt (50 kg) sack of cement in front of them for 3 or 4 hours, manhandling it in and out of a car and carting it up and down a few flights of stairs. This, they agree, would cripple them. Yet this is the size of the excess baggage they carry with them from morn to night every day! No wonder their back muscles tire, their ligaments grow strained and their spinal joints become the site of degenerative change. Often I am tempted to send these patients away, with an invitation to come back when they have shed their excess poundage. I don't do this because I appreciate how difficult it is for fat folk to change their pattern of exercising and eating and I know that it is often possible to relieve their pains without diminishing their waistlines. But there is no doubt that people who are overweight greatly increase their risk of suffering back pains and sciatica. You cannot be as fit as a fiddle when you are shaped like a double bass.

For one thing, overweight people invariably adopt a very poor posture. They carry their excess avoirdupois in front of them, which throws their backs into an uncomfortable hollow. This overstretches certain of the spinal ligaments and reduces the diameter of the foramen through which the spinal nerves emerge, increasing the risk of nerve-root compression. The constant extension of the spine also throws the weight of the trunk on to the posterior vertebral joints, making them more prone to injury and long-term degenerative change. Pregnant women are prone to backache because they carry the weight of their babies in front of them. This forces their spines into a painful backward bend. Exactly the same is true of the bow-fronted beer-drinker, only he is not so easily delivered of his burden!

People with heavy, protuberant abdomens also place an additional strain on their spinal muscles. When we bend, stretch, lift or carry, the body pivots about a fulcrum which is roughly placed in the centre of the intervertebral discs. If we carry a shopping basket in our right hand, the muscles on the left side of the spine contract to prevent us veering to the right. In the same way, if we put on an ounce of abdominal fat, our back muscles make an automatic adjustment, tensing just that little bit more to keep our bodies in balance and prevent us pitching forwards. The effort they make in this case is considerably more than might be expected, owing to the leverages involved. The adipose spare tyre we acquire is situated about ten times further from the spine's pivotal point than the back muscles themselves. This exerts the leverage effect of a crowbar, with the result that every pound (0.45 kg) of surplus belly fat we carry causes a 10 lb (4.5 kg) rise in the strain on the back. So the person who is 4 stone (25.5 kg) overweight is constantly subjecting their back to an excess loading of a quarter of a ton (254 kg)! Anyone who suffers back pain or sciatica has a very good reason to keep slim. Even 1 lb (0.45 kg) of excess weight should be avoided. It is not difficult these days to obtain tables showing standard weights for various heights but these are not always the most accurate guide of optimum body weight. Here are three more accurate ways of assessing whether or not you are carrying excess weight:

☆ *Appearance*   Strip off in front of a mirror and take a good, full frontal look at yourself. Have you still got a youthful figure? Are there any signs of a middle-aged spread, flabbiness around the thighs or maybe the suggestion of a double chin? If so, you are certainly overweight.

☆ *Weight At Maturity*   If you can remember the weight you were at 25 years old, and you were fit and active at that time, this can safely be taken as your optimum weight. Any weight which you have accumulated since then is almost certainly fat, unless you have taken up some strenuous sport or physical activity which has increased your muscle bulk.

☆ *Skin-Fold Measurement*   This is the most accurate way of discovering whether or not you are overweight. Approximately half our body fat is deposited within the skin, so it is possible to assess the size of the body's fat stores by measuring the thickness of the skin. If you pinch your skin between thumb and forefinger, you can get a good idea of the size of your personal fat stores. To do the job thoroughly the measurement should be made with a micrometer or pair of specially designed skin-fold calipers. Pinch the skin midway between your navel and groin. You are overweight if the fold measures more than ¾ in (19 mm) in the case of a man (usually the thickness of a man's little finger) and about 1 in (27 mm) for women (which is normally the thickness of a woman's thumb).

If you find you are overweight by any or all of these tests, take the strain off your back by reducing the load on your stomach. You can do this if you choose by following any Calorie-controlled diet but a far better way to slim is to step up your level of exercise. People put on weight as they grow older, not because they consume more food but because they decrease their level of exercise. This is the reason for the ubiquitous middle-aged spread. Surveys show that many fat adults actually eat less than their slim neighbours. They grow obese only because they lead excessively sedentary lives. Their primary sin is not gluttony but sloth.

The average sedentary individual gets a little less active as he ages and, as a result, puts on about 1 lb (0.45 kg) of surplus weight a year once he passes the age of 25 years. That increase in weight could be checked by taking a trifle more exercise, which need amount to no more than 3 minutes' extra walking a day. This is the simplest way to *keep* slim and the most satisfactory way to *get* slim. Take an extra half-hour's stroll a day and you will burn up 12 lb (5.4 kg) of fat by the end of a year. Have a half-hour's swim three times a week and you will shed 14 lb (6.4 kg) a year. Choose whatever form of exercise you fancy, carry it out regularly, and you will find the pounds melting away. In the process, you will lessen the strain on your back, improve the strength of your trunk and leg muscles and increase the flexibility of your hips and spine.

VERDICT   A valuable preventive measure for all back-sufferers.

4 Hydraulic Support

It is no coincidence that victims of back pain often have exceedingly weak abdominal muscles and are unable to carry out the screening test described on page 16, because the stomach muscles are one of the back's major supports. When the muscles of the abdominal wall are weak, the spine is more prone to extension injuries, postural fatigue and lifting strains. These are almost certainly the most neglected muscles in the entire body and the ones most liable to become flabby from disuse atrophy. The middle-aged spread which so many people acquire with advancing years is not just an accumulation of unwanted fat; the unsightly bulge they carry before them is generally also due to a loss of muscle tone and consequent belly sag. Two thousand years ago, Hippocrates propounded the 'Law of Use' which states: 'That which is used develops. That which is not used wastes away'. This is particularly obvious in the case of the abdominal muscles, which are so under-employed in the life of the average sedentary adult today that they waste away much faster than any other muscle group in the body. Tests carried out at the Department of Mechanical and Aerospace Engineering, Rutgers University, reveal that the strength of the abdominal muscles declines quite rapidly from the age of 30 years onwards. This decline is part of the price we pay for our sedentary way of life and is one of the reasons why our generation is so prone to spinal strain.

The abdominal muscles protect the spine in three main ways. In the first place, they act as guy ropes to hold the front of the spine in place. In this function, they are supported by the two iliopsoas muscles, which run along the inside of the spine from lumbar vertebrae to hip bone. The spine is well supplied with muscles to its rear but has little more than the power of the abdominal and iliopsoas muscles to protect its anterior aspect. It is these muscles which actively bend the trunk forward and these muscles which cushion the impact of backward bending strains. If these muscles are allowed to grow weak, the joints and ligaments of the back are more likely to be damaged when weights are lifted above the head – in backward falls or when limbo dancing! Strangely enough, most schedules of back-rehabilitation exercises emphasize the strengthening of the erector spinae muscles, which *extend* the back, but often overlook the needs of the abdominal muscles, which serve the equally vital function of *flexing* the trunk. Yet laboratory tests show that the spine's little-used flexor muscles are generally only about half a strong as the powerful extensor muscles, which are frequently brought into play to resist the downward pull of gravity. Moreover, when ergonomic tests are carried out on human volunteers placed in a rocking-chair dynamometer, which enables them to bend their trunks backwards and forwards against the resistance of spring-loaded bars, it is found that the spine's flexor muscles are not only weaker than their antagonists, but also far more quick to tire.

The second important function of the abdominal muscles, the prevention of postural droop, will not be considered here, since it is dealt with in detail on page 31. The third way in which the abdominal muscles give protection to the spine is of equal importance and yet little understood. The abdomen forms an enclosed cavity, bounded by the pelvic basin below, the spine behind, the dome-shaped diaphragm muscle above and the muscles which form the abdominal wall in front. Inside are a collection of tubes and visceral organs, which vary in

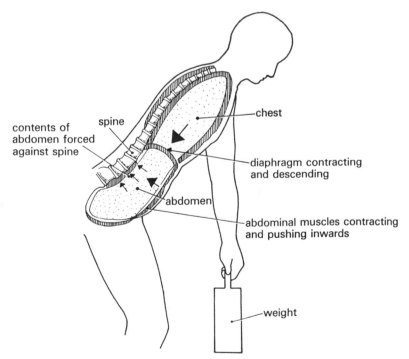

Figure 4 The abdominal buoyancy bag.

structure but have one biological feature in common, they are 80–90 per cent water. This means that they are virtually incompressible. When we breathe in, the diaphragm descends. Since the abdominal contents cannot be compressed, and they cannot deform the bony spine and pelvis, there is only one direction in which they can go and that is forwards. So, with every inspiration we make, there is an automatic and inevitable relaxation and forward displacement of the abdominal wall. It is as if we had a rugby ball, inflated with water, lodged within our bellies. When we take a deep inspiration, the diaphragm descends to make way for the expansion of the lungs. This forces the ball downwards and causes the tummy wall to bulge. If we need to cough, to clear our lungs of phlegm or dust particles, we make a sharp contraction of the abdominal wall. This drives the ball upwards against the diaphragm, causing a sudden expulsion of air from the lungs. Something similar happens when we lift a heavy weight. In this instance, both the diaphragm and the abdominal wall contract together. This squeezes the ball against the vertebral column, acting rather like the buoyancy bags used to raise sunken ships (see Figure 4).

This hydraulic device provides important support for the spine during sudden explosive efforts, as has been scientifically demonstrated in recent years. Initially, the pressure fluctuations within the abdomen were measured by introducing, through the rectum, a balloon attached to a fine catheter tube. Now a far more sophisticated technique is used. Volunteers swallow a little lozenge, which contains a tiny pressure transducer and miniature radio transmitter. With this device, it is possible to record the pressure changes within the abdominal cavity from moment to moment. Experiments with this ingenious radio pill show that the abdominal pressure mounts whenever the spine is involved in lifting strains. If the tummy muscles are strong, a high pressure can be built up within the abdominal cavity, providing powerful hydraulic

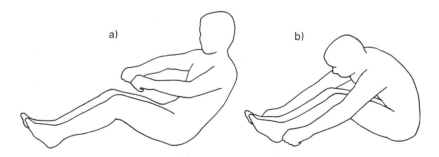

Figure 5 Rowing exercise: a) midway position b) full stretch.

support for the spine. If the tummy muscles are weak, the fluid-filled bag within the abdomen slides forward under pressure and gives about as much support to the back as a deflating whoopee cushion.

In the past, a strong, flat tummy was accepted as a cosmetic asset; now it must be regarded as a biomechanical necessity. To cultivate it, make a point of keeping the tummy muscles in regular use. From time to time, retract the abdominal wall and try and pin your navel to your spine. This is a simple exercise that can be performed at odd moments during the day: when driving a car, watching television or standing in the check-out queue at the supermarket. Two further strengthening exercises should be carried out every day.

☆ *Rowing* Lie flat on the floor with arms by your side, then carry out a rowing action with your arms and legs, bending the knees towards the chest and at the same time raising the trunk and stretching the hands to touch the feet. Return to the starting position and repeat ten times, or until you feel your stomach muscles beginning to ache (see Figure 5).

☆ *Trunk Twists* Sit on the floor with your legs stretched out in front of you and arms clasped behind your neck. Now twist to the left and try to place your right elbow on your left knee. Then twist in the opposite direction, attempting once more to put your elbow on your knee (see Figure 6). Repeat this entire sequence ten times. This exercise strengthens the lateral abdominal muscles, which play a vital role in maintaining the efficiency of the thoracolumbar fascial brace, described in the chapter which follows.

VERDICT Developing your abdominal muscles will give you a natural wrap-round corset, which will improve your posture and protect your spine from strain. You will also look better without that unsightly tummy bulge, a useful bonus when next it is time to don a bathing suit!

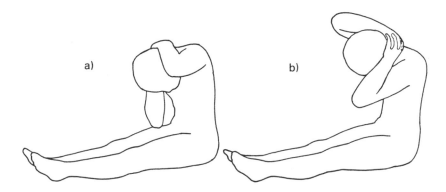

Figure 6 Trunk twists: a)rotating to the left b) rotating to the right.

5 The Fascial Brace

The base of the spine is a weak link in our skeletal chain for a number of biomechanical reasons. One factor in particular increases its vulnerability: it marks the junction between a mobile spine and a relatively rigid pelvis. Every time we twist and turn, straighten and stoop, we impart a tiny tug at the lumbosacral junction, the place where the last segment of our jointed vertebral chain is attached to the fixed sacral bone. During the course of a day, we must execute this action several hundred times. Nearly every movement we make – bending down to put on our shoes, reaching up to close a window, twisting round to pick up the telephone – either starts or ends at the base of the spine. Anyone who has had a bad back will appreciate the truth of this statement. In this condition, even the gentle action of lifting the head from the pillow can impart a painful pull at the base of the spine, while a stumble over a loose rug can give the lumbosacral junction an agonising yank. These repeated jars and jerks may be inconsequential in themselves but have a cumulative effect something akin to metal fatigue. One simple way of breaking a piece of wire is to place it in a vice and bend it rapidly backwards and forwards. Given this treatment, even the toughest of metals will show signs of stress fatigue and will eventually fracture at the point where it is fixed to the vice. The spine is subjected to exactly the same stresses, not throughout its length, where it has a high degree of flexibility, but at the point where it is clamped into the pelvis.

The early electric clothes-irons suffered a similar fate. After a few months use, their flexes cracked, always at the same point – where they were inserted into the plug at the back of the iron. This made rewiring a regular necessity until an unknown inventor thought of a cunning solution. He developed a flexible wire sleeve to protect the vulnerable portion of the flex. This was tightly wound, and therefore least flexible, where the flex was attached to the iron, and became progressively less rigid as the coil travelled away from the iron. This helped to spread the strain on the wire so that the bending took place gradually over a distance of about 4 in (10 cm), rather than abruptly at one fixed point.

This seemed a totally novel solution to a tricky problem but, in fact,

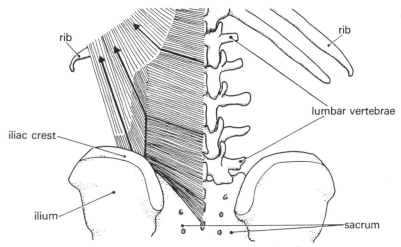

Figure 7 Thoracolumbar fascia. The arrows show the line of muscle pull.

the technique had been in use for at least ¾ million years, or since Man evolved. The assumption of the erect posture greatly increased the strain on the base of the spine and introduced it to the insidious effect of whiplash fatigue. To counteract this hazard, early Man developed a protective brace very similar to that used to shield the flex of modern irons. This sheath, instead of being made of wire, rubber or plastic, was made of fascia, stout sheets of connective tissue which the body uses to support, bind and pack its various parts. This sleeve, known to doctors as the thoracolumbar fascia, is exceedingly strong. Tests show that it is capable of taking a load of over 2,000 lb (over 900 kg) without breaking. It runs in three layers, which are attached below to the sacrum, the crest of the pelvis and the knobs or spinous processes at the back of each lumbar vertebrae (see Figure 7). From here, the fibres run upwards and outwards to provide attachments to three major muscles, two being part of the abdominal muscle group, the other being the powerful latissimus dorsi muscle which runs under each arm and which, when well developed, helps to give body-builders their envied tapered torsos.

The design of this fascial sleeve is similar to that on a clothes-iron, in that its fibres are at their toughest and densest at the point of maximum strain, the lumbosacral joint. From here, they grow progressively weaker and more sparse as they spread upwards and outwards. This arrangement helps to cushion the base of the spine from the effect of sudden bends and twists. The fascial sleeve is also a major support for the spine during bending. This has been proved by experiments on corpses for, if the tension on the thoracolumbar fascia is increased by giving it an outward pull, the lumbosacral joint is automatically thrown into extension. This shows that its function in life is to control excessive bending.

27

There is one further feature of the back's fascial sleeve which makes it distinctly superior to the supportive cuff surrounding the flex of an iron – its tension can be varied. If the pull of the latissimus dorsi and abdominal muscles is decreased, the tension in the thoracolumbar fascia is lessened. This is useful when maximum spinal flexibility is desired. Conversely, when the muscular guy ropes are contracted, the tension of the fascial sheath is increased. This is invaluable when performing heavy manual work. Trials carried out at the Bio-Engineering Centre, Wayne State University, have confirmed that the latissimus dorsi muscles contract during lifting, as do the two abdominal muscles attached to the fascial sheath.

These findings have two important practical conclusions. The first is that the back is strengthened by exercises which develop the power of the lattissimus dorsi and abdominal muscles. The strengthening of the abdominal muscles has been dealt with in the last chapter (see page 25) but the latissimus dorsi muscles need emphasis for they are frequently neglected in keep-fit programmes. Exercises to strengthen the latissimus dorsi muscles demand a place in any comprehensive schedule of back-strengthening exercises. Since a prime function of the latissimus dorsi muscles is to draw the arms towards the trunk, they can be developed by performing 'chin-ups'. This is a popular military exercise, which is included in most tests of physical fitness. The instructions are quite simple: hang from a bar and then bend both arms until your chin touches the bar. Repeat twelve times or until you reach the point of fatigue. As this is a strenuous exercise, it is better suited for athletes and army recruits than for the majority of sufferers from back pain. A gentler alternative is to place both hands on the hips with the elbows out and then to press downwards and inwards as if trying to squeeze 40-in (102 cm) hips into a pair of size 10 jeans! This exercise, which is also excellent for firming the bust, should be performed several times a day.

The second practical lesson to be learned is that the greater the rigidity of the pelvis, the greater the strain on the lumbosacral joint. When manhandling loads, shifting furniture or sawing wood, it is important to keep the hips and knees as relaxed and flexible as possible. In this way, some of the force is dissipated in movement of the legs rather than focussed on the base of the spine. People with stiff hamstring muscles are particularly prone to damage their backs because they quickly come to the end of their range of hip-joint movement when they bend. As a result, they are forced to make more pivotal use of their lumbosacral joints. The same applies to abnormal tightness elsewhere in the pelvic region. If the rotation of the hip joint is limited by shortening of the joint capsules or tightness of the rotator muscles (see page 64), the base of the spine is forced to bear a greater share of the strain whenever twisting movements are made. In the same way, when there is excessive tightness in the lateral stabilisers of the hip, the lumbosacral joint is subjected to additional strain during side-bending movements, such as occur when climbing up and down stairs. This is particularly obvious when the movements of the hip joints are grossly restricted by osteo-arthritis. Then even simple everyday movements, like walking, rolling out of bed, putting on shoes, or rising from a chair, impose a major strain on the base of the spine. This is why patients with stiff, arthritic hips often complain more of the pain in their backs than the ache in their legs. Restoring the movement of their hips, by giving them artificial joint replacements, is often sufficient to ease their lumbago without applying any treatment whatsoever to the spine itself.

One of the great advantages of yoga exercises is that they improve the flexibility of the legs and upper trunk and, in so doing, reduce the strain on the vulnerable lumbosacral joint.

VERDICT *Time spent strengthening the muscles which support the thoracolumbar fascia is never wasted. Exercises which maintain the mobility of the hip joints are also well rewarded, for both measures reduce the overall strain on the lumbosacral joint, which is the weakest link in the spine's skeletal chain.*

6 We Stoop, But Not To Conquer

Man is the only creature which has to think about its posture. Immediately after birth, a foal will struggle to its feet and take a few faltering steps and a lamb will stumble after its mother in search of food. Not so the human child, which takes months of patient, and often painful, endeavour before it finally 'finds its feet'. This is part of the price we pay for having assumed the upright posture.

This stance has greatly increased our potential and considerably magnified our physical problems, not least of which is the difficulty of maintaining the erect position against the constant downward pull of gravity. This is a complex mechanical task which no other animal has to tackle and which few human beings perform satisfactorily. When two physiotherapists from the Children's Hospital School in Baltimore examined the posture of 12,000 people, both children and adults, they found practically no one who was in ideal postural balance. Many were unaware of their postural faults and were unwittingly suffering unnecessary tiredness and strain because of their poor carriage. Others were suffering symptoms – backache, fibrositis and tension headaches – which were the direct consequence of their poor body mechanics.

Poor posture is a common, and generally easily remedied, cause of back pain. One of the commonest postural faults is an increase in the curvatures of the spine. At birth, our spines are held in a single backward curve, as are those of monkeys and apes. The uniqueness of the human spine appears in early infancy, when we learn to stand upright. First a reverse curve appears in the neck as we master the art of holding the head erect; then a hollow appears in the lumbar spine as we struggle to stand on our feet. This sequence of hollows and humps enable us to hold our bodies erect and increases both the flexibility and strength of the spine. (It has been estimated that providing the spine with spring-like joints and curves enables it to withstand shocks 100 times more efficiently than if the vertebrae were placed directly one on top of the other and cushioned only by their intervening discs.) From the point of view of mechanical stability, it would appear much more sensible to place the vertebrae, like building blocks, one directly on top of the other, so that

30

the weight of the body passes directly through the skeleton with no risk of postural deformation. As it is, there is a constant tendency for the curves to be exaggerated by the downward pull of gravity. Nowhere is this more obvious than in the lumbar spine, which is often thrown into a pronounced hollow. In this position of extreme backward bending, ligaments are placed on full stretch and the joints at the back of the vertebrae are forced to carry more than their fair share of the work load. This makes them prone to injury and degenerative change.

Several things contribute to the development of an exaggerated lumbar curve, as can be seen in Figure 8. An abdomen overloaded with superfluous fat will shift the weight of the body forward and force the spine to make a compensatory backward curve. Heavy, pendulous breasts or a drooping head will have exactly the same effect. Sheer laziness may also cause a forward shift of the body weight, so that the body adopts a characteristic slouching posture with head slumped, shoulders drooped and belly bulging forward. If the tummy muscles are allowed to become slack, this increases the tendency for the lumbar spine to arch, as does any stiffness in the posterior spinal muscles.

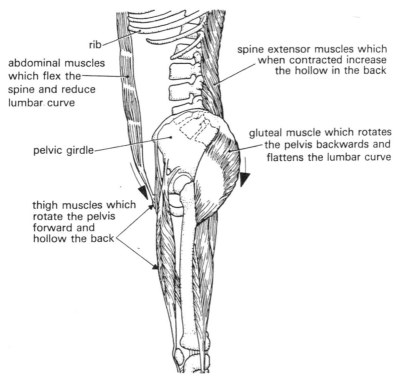

Figure 8 The lumbar curve.

There is one simple way of telling whether or not you are suffering from an excess curvature of the spine. Strip off to your underclothes and stand with your back to a wall and your heels 4 in (10 cm) from the skirting board. In this position, the head, shoulder blades and seat should make easy contact with the wall, leaving a gap in the small of the back which is just deep enough to accommodate the flat of your hand. Any exaggeration in these curves will leave your head thrust forward out of contact with the wall, the shoulders rounded and the lumbar region of the back arched so excessively that it will contain not just the flat of your hand but also the closed fist, as shown in Figure 9. To correct this common postural fault:

☆ Get rid of any surplus weight.
☆ Strengthen your abdominal muscles, as outlined on page 25.
☆ Stretch out the structures which may be holding your back in a rigid

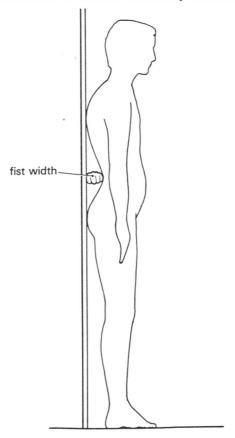

fist width

Figure 9 *Bad posture showing an exaggeration of the spinal curve.*

arch by performing loosening exercise 3 on page 71.

☆ Make a conscious effort to stand and walk tall, imagining that you are a puppet being lifted upward by your central string or a bearer carrying a heavy weight upon your head.

☆ Try to keep the major weight masses of your body – head, chest, pelvis and thighs – directly in line, one above the other, with the centre of gravity of your body falling nearer to your heel than the forepart of your foot. In this position, you will minimise the strain on your back and reduce the work load on your body's anti-gravity muscles.

While examining your posture, it is advisable to look as well for any unwanted lateral curves. Ideally the spine should be plumb-line straight from skull to pelvis but often it takes a deviation to the side. These lateral curves can be detected by standing in front of a full-length mirror, again in underclothes. If in this position you notice that one shoulder is lower than the other, one hip more prominent than its fellow, the head tilted slightly to one side, or the waist crease more marked on one side of the body, the chances are that you have a lateral curvature of the spine, or scoliosis (see Figure 10). Standing tall can help to minimise these lateral curves, as was demonstrated by a trial which revealed that correcting an exaggerated lumbar curve was just as effective in correcting lateral curvature as wearing a spinal brace. Providing these sideways kinks are not too marked, they rarely give rise to symptoms and can be improved by exercises which improve the posture and strengthen the spine's supporting muscles. If the deformities are marked, and accompanied by rotation of the spine which distorts the rib cage, it is advisable to seek specialist medical help.

In addition to these measures, there is one tip which can lessen the impact of postural deformities of all degrees and kinds: never stand still a moment longer than you need. One reason why backache is so rare among Third World peoples is that they rarely stand in one place. If they are watching over a cooking pot, they will sit cross-legged in front of the fire rather than stand. If they are waiting for the daily visit of the village bus, they will squat on their haunches rather than stand in a queue. Londoners are often amazed to see wealthy Arab ladies sitting on the pavement outside Harrods waiting for their chauffeur-driven Rolls to take them and their purchases back to their penthouse suites. This, in the eyes of an orthodoxly brought-up Briton, is bizarre behaviour, and yet it is a sensible way of resting and lessening the postural strain on the back, even if the pavement is a trifle grubby. In the West, we spend far too long standing still, at cocktail parties, in supermarket check-out queues and while ironing and cooking, preparing food, watching games and waiting for buses and trains. This is never a salutary exercise.

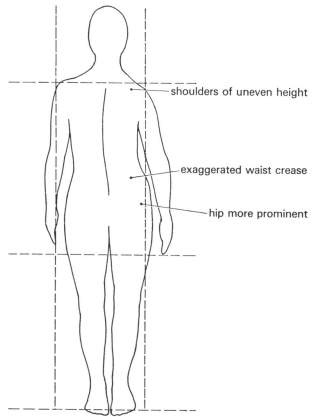

shoulders of uneven height

exaggerated waist crease

hip more prominent

Figure 10 Lateral curvature of the spine.

Periods of standing should be kept to a minimum and interspersed, whenever possible, with short bouts of movement to relieve the strain on the spinal ligaments. Even if it may seem at times a trifle eccentric, it pays to observe the old Turkish proverb: 'Never stand up when you can sit down; never sit down when you can lie down'.

VERDICT Backache is often aggravated by the postural strain of standing, so it is always advisable to learn to stand well and to make a practice of reducing spells of standing to an absolute minimum.

7 Lopsided Limbs

Equality is the political idealist's dream, but it is not our birthright, as every doctor knows. Even our two sides differ. Chiropodists note that we generally have one foot broader than its partner. Photographers seem convinced that we invariably have one side of our face which is more photogenic than the other. In eight out of ten cases, our right shoulder drops lower than the left. A less-recognized asymmetry is that we often walk about on legs of unequal length.

A short while ago, doctors from the University of Copenhagen studied the posture of a large proportion of the adult population of Glostrup, a suburb of Copenhagen. They found that virtually 29 per cent of the people studied had a significant difference in the length of their legs, measuring ½ in (1 cm) or more. For some odd reason, it was the left leg which was generally the shorter of the two, in the ratio of roughly 5:3. When they singled out the people suffering from back pain, they found that the incidence of anisomelia, the medical term for leg-length discrepancy, rose to 46 per cent. Previous studies in the UK showed that anisomelia was twice as common in people with back pain as in those without. Obviously having legs of differing length is a structural disadvantage for it throws the pelvis out of kilter and forces the spine to adopt a lateral curve to maintain the postural balance. If the hips and spine are mobile, this may cause no discomfort whatsoever. I have examined patients with leg-length differences of ½ in (1 cm) or more who have compensated so well for their anatomical discrepancy that they have had no sign of back trouble throughout their lives until they reached maybe their 60s or 70s, when the compensation broke down and they started to suffer spinal pain. Others, with no greater difference, have suffered chronic back pains from their early teens. In them, the structural asymmetry causes postural strain from the outset, especially when they are standing. Later, they are likely to suffer degenerative changes in their spines. This was confirmed by a recent X-ray study of patients with chronic back pain. The subjects were divided into two groups: one with leg-length discrepancies, the others without. Comparison afterwards showed that degenerative changes of the spine – the development of bony spurs and wedge-shaped vertebrae – were more likely to be found in the group of patients showing significant degrees of anisomelia. Obviously it is advisable to check the development of these permanent changes before they occur if it is humanly possible, even at a stage before symptoms start to occur.

Patients often ask the obvious question: 'Why do legs grow to different lengths?' Sometimes it is possible to give an easy explanation. Legs occasionally become shorter after they have been fractured. The remodelling of the bones which occurs with disorders such as rickets, Paget's disease or osteo-arthritis of the hip can also result in shortening of the affected leg. I have also known one leg to grow longer than its fellow when it has been the site of chronic osteomyelitis but, more often than not, there is no rational explanation for anisomelia. From the ages of 1–20 years, the limbs grow 2 ft (60 cm) or more in length, from six main growing centres, known as epiphyses. It takes only a slight slow-down in the activity of one of these centres, or an acceleration of another, to produce a difference in leg lengths. Just a 1 per cent per annum variation in the rate of activity of these centres could produce a significant difference in the leg lengths by the time bone growth comes to an end. The truly remarkable thing, therefore, is not that legs sometimes grow to different lengths but that they are so often such a perfect match!

At one time, little help was given to people with leg-length discrepancies, except to advise them to live on the side of a mountain! Now they can be assisted in two main ways. Firstly, they are encouraged to maintain the fullest possible mobility of their hips and spine, so that their bodies can assume a slightly asymmetrical posture without strain. Secondly, when it is appropriate, they can be fitted with heel lifts of an appropriate height to balance the length of their legs.

But treatment cannot proceed until an accurate diagnosis is made. Differences in leg lengths can generally be detected on a routine standing postural examination. Confirmation of the discrepancy is generally made with a tape measure when the subjects are lying on their backs on an examination couch, each leg being measured from the bony knob on the front of the pelvis to the lower limit of the inner ankle bone. The difference in these two measurements gives some indication of the degree of anisomelia. A more accurate assessment can be obtained by taking a standing pelvic X-ray, when the difference in the heights of the two hip bones can be measured directly on the X-ray plate.

Sometimes the subjects themselves are vaguely aware that the lower part of their bodies is out of kilter. They may notice that, when they are standing, one hip is higher than the other. Ladies may find that the hems of their skirts do not fall evenly, or that when they are walking in the rain they splash one leg more than its partner. Others may observe that they come down more heavily on one heel than the other when they walk, or that they wear out the sole of one shoe before its fellow. An even more characteristic symptom of anisomelia is a rolling gait. For ages, it was thought that the badger had longer legs on one side of its body than the other because it wobbled from side to side as it walked. According to the seventeenth-century writer Sir Thomas Browne, this was not a folk myth since the theory was upheld by experts 'who have opportunity to behold and hunt' the badger. In fact, badgers generally have well-matched limbs, but a similar rolling gait is seen in human beings who exhibit leg-length discrepancies. With them, the telltale sign is an exaggerated dipping of the shoulders as they walk, which is most marked on the side of the short leg.

If you think you might have a leg-length discrepancy, strip off and examine yourself in front of a full-length mirror, both standing and sitting. As you stand, you might notice that your hips and shoulders are on different levels. It is easier to spot the difference in hip heights if you rest your hands at waist level on the crests of the pelvis, with palms flat and facing directly downwards. If the asymmetry in the positioning of the shoulders and hips is caused by an inequality of leg lengths, it will disappear the moment you sit down (providing your spine is still mobile and not fixed in a long-standing compensatory lateral curve). If you are lop-sided when you stand, try correcting the asymmetry by placing a slim paperback book or pamphlet under the heel of what appears to be your short leg. If this levels your hips and shoulders, it is highly likely that you have a leg-length discrepancy. The problem now is what action to take. The safest measure is to seek the advice of someone with a specialist knowledge of back problems – doctor, osteopath, chiropractor, physiotherapist or physical medicine consultant. They *might* advise you to have a heel lift fitted to your shoe to correct your postural imbalance and ease your spinal pain.

If you are an intrepid do-it-yourself adventurer, you may be tempted to take this step without medical guidance. This has certain inherent risks. In the first place, it can be as harmful to overcorrect a leg-length discrepancy as to leave it untreated. (For this reason, it is generally advisable to apply a lift which only partially corrects the discrepancy.) The use of heel lifts can also be a disadvantage in older people, in whom the body has adapted so fully to the postural imbalance that it cannot accept any attempt at reverse correction. More serious problems can arise when the postural imbalance is accompanied by sciatic pain. In cases of anisomelia, sciatic pain normally travels down the long leg, for the simple reason that the lumbar spine is generally forced to bend towards this side to maintain balance and this increases the pressure on the roots of the sciatic nerve. But, just occasionally, sciatic pain will travel down the short leg. In these cases, the discomfort is normally made worse by wearing a heel lift on the shortened side.

Self treatment can present problems, therefore, but can be attempted if you don't mind risking a temporary exacerbation of your pain. To assess the degree of your leg-length difference, stand erect in front of a mirror, with knees straight, and slip wedges of paper under your heel until you find a thickness that almost balances the level of your hips and shoulders. This is the height of lift adjustment you need. Take this measurement to a shoe repairer, together with a pair of shoes that can be discarded if your experiment in remedial orthoptics fails, and ask him to make the necessary correction. Leave the mechanics to him. He might find it easier to make the adjustment by paring a little off the height of one heel and adding a little to the height of the other. This makes the alteration less conspicuous and less likely to disturb the balance of the shoe. Then give these shoes a therapeutic trial for a few days, especially when you have to do a lot of standing. If you find that your back tires less readily when wearing the lift, you can adopt this as a permanent prophylactic measure with some confidence.

VERDICT Discrepancies in leg lengths are a common contributory cause of postural back pain. They can generally be corrected by making an appropriate adjustment to the height of your heels. This measure should be carried out under the direction of a specialist, but can be instigated by the layman providing:

☆ *You carry out the tests described earlier to ensure that you do exhibit a genuine difference in leg lengths.*
☆ *Corrections are limited to a maximum height of ¾ in (1.9 cm).*
☆ *No attempt is made to correct for the full discrepancy in leg lengths.*
☆ *Heel lifts are used for a trial period before they are accepted as a permanent measure.*
☆ *Heel lifts are discarded if they show a tendency to aggravate back or leg pain.*

8 The Torture Chair

Whenever mention is made of good and bad posture, we invariably assume that the reference is made to the way in which we stand. Yet we adopt a wide variety of postures during the day, such as lying, sitting, standing and bending over work surfaces, and the least common of these is almost certainly the erect, standing position. Most of our waking life is spent in a chair, for this is the age of home sedentarians. Most city workers get up from their breakfast table only to take a seat in a bus, car or train to travel to work. For the remainder of the day they are ensconced behind an office desk. Then, when the day's work is done, they are whisked home to spend their leisure hours watching television from the comfort of a fireside chair. Most of the day is spent in chairs of invariably poor design, often uncomfortably slumped. This is a major cause of postural strain and back pain.

Anatomists are convinced that we have not yet adapted to the erect standing posture which we assumed some 800,000 years ago. What chance can we have had, then, to adapt to the erect sitting posture, which we assumed no more than 5,000 years ago? Occupations that involve prolonged spells of sitting generally carry a high incidence of back pain. A survey of desk workers showed that many experienced skeletal pain: 16 per cent in their seats; 19 per cent in their thighs; 24 per cent in their neck and shoulders and a massive 57 per cent in their lumbar spines. A similar situation exists among airline pilots, according to a survey carried out by BALPA, the British pilots' union. This revealed that 62 per cent of commercial pilots suffered backache, which had been the cause of sickness absenteeism in one in three. One interesting finding of the study was that half the pilots who had trouble in the air did not suffer on the ground. This is possibly because their spells of sitting were shorter and more regularly punctuated by movements about the house, and also no doubt because they were less tense when they were off-duty than when they were flying. The survey also revealed that pilots often padded their cockpit seats with paperback books or old socks to provide better support for their lumbar spines. Sometimes they were even forced to stuff their left arm into the hollow of their backs, preferring to fly one-handed than continue to suffer postural strain!

Ergonomists are by now well aware of this particular occupational hazard and it is claimed that the British Aircraft Corporation spent £350 million designing special posture-seating for their Concorde crews. Similar extravagant sums have been spent on designing other specialised seating.

Tests show that the pressure on the lumbar discs is 43 per cent higher in the sitting position than when standing. This is because more weight is brought to bear on the discs and no doubt also because the abdominal muscles relax and so cease to maintain the upward lift of the abdominal buoyancy bag (see page 23). This increased pressure may cause degenerated discs to bulge and throw more pressure on the nerve roots. But there is another reason why sitting predisposes to back strain, which is likely to be of far greater practical significance. Radiological studies have shown that, in the slumped sitting position, the lower two lumbar vertebrae are tipped forward as far as they can go. This means that, for as long as we slump in a chair, we are subjecting the ligaments of our lower back to constant stretch. This they can accept for a brief while, particularly if the surrounding muscles contract to give them protective protective support, but eventually fatigue sets in and the ligaments start to suffer from the unrelieved strain. This extreme position causes pain, just as it would if we spent a long while driving or beinding over a flower-bed. From the point of view of the positioning of the lumbar vertebrae, there is no difference between the extreme flexion experienced when driving a car in a slumped sitting position and the forward bending encountered when holding the trunk in a jack-knifed position. This is

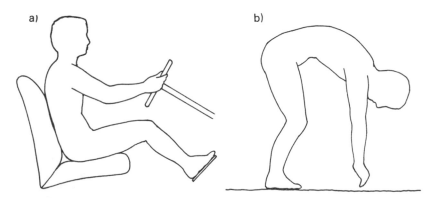

Figure 11 Postural strain: a) driving in the slumped sitting position b) weeding the garden (the same posture rotated through an angle of approximately 90°).

clearly shown in Figure 11, which depicts a man driving a car and weeding the garden but which is merely the same silhouette rotated through an angle of 90°. This explains why 3 hours' sitting in a bad position often produces as much ligament strain in the base of the spine as a morning weeding the garden.

One way of overcoming this postural strain is to sit in chairs or car seats which have a firm lumbar support, to prevent the spine from slumping into a fully flexed position. This is generally possible in adjustable typing chairs but can rarely be achieved in the plush chairs favoured by senior executives or in the general range of fireside chairs, which are about as resilient as cream-filled meringues. For some unaccountable reason, furniture manufacturers seem to be filled with flights of fancy the moment they come to create a chair. As a result, it is possible now to sit in sacks filled with polystyrene granules, on inflatable plastic chairs, glass-fibre eggshells or in hammock-like constructions of chrome tubing and canvas webbing. Not so long ago, a young architect realized that he had developed backache only since his office was re-equipped with ultra-modern furniture. On closer investigation, he discovered that he had been sitting on what was intended to be a wastepaper basket! This may be an apocryphal tale but it does emphasize the point that most avant-garde chair design today is based on principles which are eye-catching rather than functional.

How is it possible to sort through this wide assortment of designs and find a chair which gives you good postural support? It is useless to accept the recommendation of friends for what suits them will almost certainly not suit you. Both at work and in the home, we should install chairs which suit our individual needs. Grouped around the fireside, there should be a father's chair and a mother's chair and individual chairs for all the other members of the family. Three-piece suites may be the delight of interior designers but they are the bêtes-noires of osteopaths and orthopaedic surgeons.

One day, no doubt, it will be possible to go into a furniture store and be measured for a chair, just as today we are measured for a suit. This will not be cheap, but then nor is the hand-tailored suit, and it will provide a more valuable service than bespoke tailoring for, while an off-the-peg suit may not fit too well, it does not cripple like a badly fitting chair. Until that happy day arrives, it will be necessary to shop around and select, by a process of trial and error, a chair that fits one's frame and does not cause backache, leg pain or numbness in the feet and thighs. The diagram (overleaf) shows the key points to look for when buying a chair (Figure 12). These key points are:

☆ A firm seat, to facilitate the regular slight shifts of posture that are

41

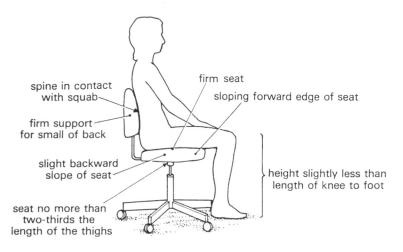

spine in contact
with squab

firm seat

sloping forward edge of seat

firm support
for small of back

slight backward
slope of seat

height slightly less than
length of knee to foot

seat no more than
two-thirds the
length of the thighs

Figure 12 Key points to look for when buying a chair.

necessary to stave off fatigue and prevent the prolonged compression of delicate tissues.

☆ A sloping forward edge to avoid compression of the veins and arteries which run above the back of the knee.

☆ A seat placed at a height from the ground which is slightly less than the length of the leg from knee to foot. This enables the feet to be firmly planted on the ground so that they take most of the weight of the thighs, thereby avoiding pressure on the soft tissues of the upper leg, which can be compressed to a third of their normal thickness in chairs of unsuitable height.

☆ A seat which is no more than two-thirds of the length of the thighs, so that the spine can be kept in contact with the squab support at the back of the chair.

☆ Firm support for the small of the back.

☆ Slight backward slope of the seat (about 7–8°) to ensure that the weight of the body does not slip forward but is pressed into the support of the chair.

If your chair or car seat does not provide adequate cushioning for your back, try using one of the many patent back supports. And, if your fireside seat or office chair is provided with arm rests, use them whenever you can, for tests show that this can ease the pressure on the back by taking up to 12 per cent of the total body weight.

But it is wrong to think only of static sitting strains. It is a basic principle of good posture that no one position of the body is ideal if maintained too long. Constant shifts of posture are necessary to stave off fatigue and prevent prolonged stretching of the spine's supporting ligaments. These fatigue-relieving movements are performed automatically when we stand and at regular intervals when we sleep but are less easily achieved when we are pinioned in a chair – unless we revert to using an old-fashioned rocking chair, which Dr Barry Wyke, director of the Royal College of Surgeons' Neurological Unit, believes is one of the finest ways of reducing the incidence of back pains in the over-40s. This opinion was shared by Dr Janet Travell who, during her days as physical medicine consultant to the White House, advised President Kennedy to install a rocking chair in his personal office suite to ease his spinal pain. 'The constantly changing position will relax your muscles and rest you', she assures back sufferers.

Some modern chairs are specially designed to permit a greater range of trunk and limb movements. A British firm has developed chairs with rubber joints. This enables the frame, seat and legs to move independently, which it is hoped will permit movements of the body to be made with minimum muscular effort. A Danish company has pioneered chairs with a tilting seat, designed by orthopaedic surgeon Dr Aage Mandel, which allow schoolchildren and office-workers to move easily from an upright position to a forwardly inclined writing position. Another notable Scandinavian development is the range of chairs created by Dr Balans, which take pressure on the knees and allow the body weight to be shifted easily from the pelvis to shins (see Figure 13)

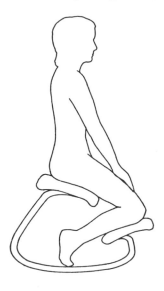

Figure 13 Balans chair.

Another school of thought suggests that we might be better off dispensing with chairs altogether. One reason why the peoples of Third World countries rarely suffer back pains is that they rarely adopt a static sedentary pose. When they rest, they either squat on their haunches or sit cross-legged on the floor. In either position, they are free to shift their weight from side to side and from front to rear, which eases the strain on the ligaments of the spine. Following their example, I have advised a number of my patients to go native during the evening and to exchange their easy chairs for a cushion on the floor. Many have found this far more comfortable for their backs.

One further safeguard is to limit the length of prolonged sitting spells, breaking up long car journeys with regular wayside halts, and interspersing extended air flights with occasional strolls up and down the gangway or long evening sojourns reading or watching TV in a chair with a tour of inspection of the garden or a trip to the kitchen to make a cup of tea.

VERDICT *Many back problems are aggravated by sedentary postural strains. These can be minimized by using chairs of sound design and by making regular shifts of posture.*

9 Driven To Despair

People without cars don't realize how lucky they are. They may enjoy the financial saving and the lessened mental strain of travelling by foot instead of by car but they are unlikely to appreciate that, as non-motorists, they are three times less likely to suffer back pain than high-mileage drivers. One explanation is that driving necessitates sitting for spells in a tense, cramped and frequently slumped position. This invites postural fatigue and low back strain.

The average driver spends nearly 2 weeks a year sitting behind the wheel of a car. If his driving position is poor, or the car seat badly designed, he is undoubtedly a high risk candidate for back pain. A short while ago, a number of motorists were asked to test-drive a popular family saloon with a notoriously poor driving seat. At the end of the trip, half complained of spinal aches and pains. Motor-car manufacturers are well aware of this problem and are endeavouring to produce seats which provide far better support for the back. In this quest, they face one major drawback: their customers are not of equal build. If they design a seat which is suitable for a slimly built lady of 5 ft 2 in (157 cm), it will not be suitable for her 6-ft (182-cm) husband and even less so for her gangling son, who may be touching 6 ft 2 in (188 cm). So they endeavour to strike a happy compromise – but no such thing exists. Furniture manufacturers and car designers have tried in the past to construct a picture of the average man and woman, only to find that the concept has no practical relevance.

Detailed measurements were taken of a group of over 4,000 people, including such dimensions as height, seat width and leg and arm length. From these measurements, a composite blue print was obtained of the mean figure. The intentions of this survey were good but the results were disastrous. The researchers set out to please everyone and ended up satisfying nobody for, at the end of their investigations, they found that not one of the 4,000 subjects fitted all the bodily dimensions of the mythical average figure. We are all individuals, in our body shape as well as in our voice and fingerprints, and the only thing car manufacturers can do to provide a universally acceptable driving position is to create driving seats which are capable of as much adjustment as a typist's chair.

It has been estimated that the seating requirements of 90 per cent of motorists could be met if driving seats had a 6-in (15-cm) range of fore-and-aft adjustment and a 4-in (10-cm) range of independent height adjustment. As it is, few small family cars have this full range of fore-and-aft adjustment and virtually none provide any independent height adjustment, merely racking up an inch or so as the seat is moved forward.

Anyone who cares for their back and spends much time motoring should pay close attention to the design of their car seat. In particular they should look for:

☆ A driving seat with a firm squab, which facilitates the small adjustments of posture which are necessary to stave off muscular fatigue and prevent prolonged ligament strain.

☆ A seat which has a wide enough range of adjustment – height, rake and distance from foot controls – to permit the adoption of a comfortable driving position. One test is to make sure that the steering wheel can be gripped in the ten-to-two position without slumping forward or taking the back away from the support of the seat. In this position, it should also be possible to depress the brake pedal fully without completely straightening the knee. (Tests show that maximum thrust can be applied to the foot pedals when the knees are bent at an angle of 140°.) If you are too tall or too short for your existing car, you may be able to adapt your driving position by fitting proprietary pedal extensions and moving the seat-runners backwards or forwards or building them up with suitable packing material. For safety's sake, these modifications should be made by qualified motor mechanics rather than with faith, hope and adhesive tape. Remember too that, if you share a car with other motorists in the family, you will almost certainly need to alter the position of the driving seat before you embark on a journey of any distance.

☆ A seat placed squarely behind the foot controls. In some cars, the brake and clutch are set at a slight angle to the seat, which keeps the spine on constant torsion.

☆ A seat which provides a firm lumbar support. This is a deficiency of expensive cars as well as cheaper family saloons. If you find yourself slumping when you drive, try fitting your car with any patent back support which proves comfortable on testing.

☆ A seat which provides a degree of lateral support to prevent the spine rolling when corners are taken. The wearing of seat belts also helps to give added stability and extra anchoring to the spine, particularly during country motoring.

Those who drive long distances, and can afford it, may find their backache eased by installing custom-built driving seats of the type made for rally drivers. Regular wayside halts can also help to break up the postural strain of driving, especially when they are accompanied by a gentle stroll or a few gymnastic exercises.

In addition to suffering prolonged postural strain, drivers are also exposed to constant vibration. This too is known to predispose to back pain. Tractor drivers frequently suffer from backache, so too do long-distance truck drivers who, according to one survey, have a risk of suffering a disc prolapse which is four times higher than average. Passengers in buses and trains are also liable to have their spines bounced up and down, with the result that those who commute more than 20 miles a day to work have double the normal risk of developing a disc injury.

In the USA, it is estimated that over 8 million workers are exposed to a level of occupational vibration that could affect their health and working efficiency, causing not only back pain but also diseases such as varicose veins, piles, hernias and 'dead finger'. In the USSR, official reports suggest that vibration disease is now the third most common cause of occupational sickness. Authorities there are particularly concerned about long-distance lorry drivers, many of whom suffer from vibration sickness, a disease characterised by back pain, headaches, nausea, indigestion and rapid fatigue.

The human body is highly sensitive to vibration. Some wavelengths stimulate the delicate nerve endings in the ear and give rise to audible sound. Others, of a slightly higher frequency, set the body's water stores trembling like jelly on a plate. This can aid the interchange of tissue fluids and facilitate the absorption of inflammatory swellings, which is why physiotherapists use ultrasonic wave therapy and whirlpool baths in the treatment of rheumatic disease. As far as the body is concerned, some vibrations are beneficial, others are harmful. Senator Ted Kennedy, for example, finds that the pain in his back is aggravated by rides in a heavily vibrating bus but soothed by spells in the whirlpool bath at his mother's mansion in West Palm Beach, Florida.

Vibrations in the 10–20 Hz waveband are liable to cause headaches, those in the 40–3,000 Hz waveband provoke circulatory changes in the hands, while those in the frequency range of 5–10 Hz tend to cause back pain. When volunteers were placed on oscillating boards, it was discovered that, if their bodies were vibrated at 4 cycles per second, a typical frequency experienced when driving, the movements of the pelvis and thorax tended to get out of phase, which placed an increased strain on their spinal muscles. At frequencies of 5 cycles per second, the vibrations were inclined to be augmented, sometimes being doubled in

47

amplitude as they travelled through the body. The manufacturers of tractors, lorries and private cars are now trying to build vehicles which avoid these dangerous and tiring vibration frequencies but it is no easy task. We owe a great debt to men like Elliott, who first introduced elliptical springs into horse-drawn carriages, and Dunlop, who invented the pneumatic tyre which made the old bone-shaker bicycles obsolete. Now we await a similar breakthrough in vehicle-chassis design. Modern road-making techniques may have made motoring smoother but they cannot entirely eliminate the humps and bumps of driving, particularly on motorways where the maintenance of a regular high speed can produce a particularly exhausting, throbbing pulse.

When it comes to motoring, there is no such thing as 'good vibes', unless they are the soothing wavelengths coming from the car radio. In practice, there are four main things which can be done to protect the spine from unnecessary vibration when driving:

☆ Choose a make of car which gives a smooth, comfortable ride. A study carried out a few years ago in the New Haven and Hartford districts of Connecticut confirmed that motorists were more prone to disc injuries than non-motorists but revealed that the hazard was less for drivers of Japanese and Swedish cars. This may relate to an earlier discovery that French, Japanese and Swedish cars tend to vibrate at lower than average frequencies, whereas American, and especially German, cars vibrate at frequencies which are more nearly approaching the 4–5 Hz waveband, which throws particular stress on the lumbar spine.

☆ Avoid driving an engine at speeds approaching its maximum revolutions. Vibrations generally grow stronger when a car is pushed towards its limits, so keep to a comfortable cruising speed and there will be less strain on the car and less wear on your personal chassis. And, if your work involves regular distance driving, do not be content with an underpowered car for, if you consistently drive a rattling shoe-box, there may come a time when it is not only your prestige that suffers a damaging jolt!

☆ Attend immediately to strange rattles and knocks. If you are mechanically illiterate, you may choose to ignore even the most ominous clanking that comes from under the bonnet in the hope that it might go away if left alone. This is invariably a mistake. Insecure engine mountings, loose universal joints, damaged propeller shafts and broken fan belts set up unnecessary vibration and can also give rise to inconvenient and expensive engine failure. All merit prompt attention.

☆ Keep car wheels in good balance. A lot of vibration experienced by drivers is transmitted via the front wheels to the steering column. It is fairly easy for manufacturers to build a balanced wheel but far less easy to produce and maintain a balanced tyre, particularly when it is subjected to irregular wear and repeated scuffing against the kerb. For this reason, it is advisable to have the wheels expertly balanced from time to time. Watch out too for any odd lumps of mud adhering to the car wheels. Just 1 oz (30 g) of dirt clinging to the rim of a wheel creates a centrifugal pull of over 6 lb (2.7 kg) at 50 mph (80 km/h), which is quite enough to throw the wheel out of balance and produce an irritating vibration.

VERDICT Numerous tests have shown that motorists have an above average chance of suffering back troubles. This risk can be reduced by adopting a sound driving posture, by eliminating unnecessary vibration and by interrupting long journeys with regular pauses for rest and gentle exercise.

10 Sleeping Sickness

We spend about a third of our lives in bed. This is the scene of some of the most meaningful events of our lives. As Guy de Maupassant wrote: 'The bed, my friend, is our whole life. It is there that we are born, it is there that we love, it is there that we die'. Beds are places charged with emotive imagery: soothing, erotic, secret, therapeutic.

Bed rest has been a favoured treatment for back pain for centuries, yet many people find their spinal aches and pains are aggravated by lying down. Some go to bed in comfort and wake up in agony. Others toss and turn throughout the night, struggling to find a position which eases their pain. A number even have their first taste of acute back pain after sleeping on an uncomfortable camp bed or put-u-up. They retire to bed with backs as straight and supple as a willow branch, and wake up with spines contorted like an old, gnarled oak.

Sleeping is a high-risk activity for the spine, particularly when the vertebral joints are stiff or the bed excessively soft. While we are asleep, our muscles relax. This gives less protection to the underlying spinal ligaments and joints, which become more vulnerable to strain, particularly if they are held for too long in an uncomfortable position. The inebriate who falls asleep on a park bench, the traveller who snatches forty winks in an aircraft seat and the exhausted worker who nods off to sleep in front of the television are all liable to musculoskeletal strains of the shoulders, neck and back. Similar strains can occur in bed if faulty positions are adopted.

Most doctors today are convinced that a good bed enhances the quality of the night's repose and helps alleviate back strain. Unfortunately there is less agreement on what actually constitutes a 'good' bed. The choice is bewildering. Our ancestors slept quite comfortably on a pile of furs or a straw-filled palliasse. Many contemporary Japanese choose to sleep on the floor on a simple woven mat or flock-filled *futon*. Sailors sleep in hammocks, tramps in doorways and trendy Californians on heated water beds. Our spines are adaptable and will accept without complaint a wide range of sleeping surfaces, providing they are firm enough to serve two important functions:

50

☆ *To permit easy movement of the body* Most people change their position twenty to sixty times a night to ease the strain on their ligaments and relieve the pressure on delicate tissues. A firm bed enables these essential postural shifts to be made with minimum effort and disturbance. Studies of Swedish lumberjacks have confirmed the importance of a resilient bed, showing that men who slept on soft mattresses tended to remain static for long periods during the night, while those who slept on a firmer surface were able to escape the risk of postural strain by changing position fifty or more times while they slept.

☆ *To prevent the spine sagging* When we sleep, the postural muscles supporting the spine relax. This means that strain is thrown on the spinal ligaments whenever the back is allowed to sag beyond a certain point. A firm bed helps to prevent this strain but it should not be so hard that it provides inadequate cushioning for the body's bony points. Nor should it be so rigid that it fails to provide snug hollows for the shoulders and pelvis, or else these prominent parts of the skeleton are thrust upwards so that the spine is kinked at the waist, as shown in Figure 14a.

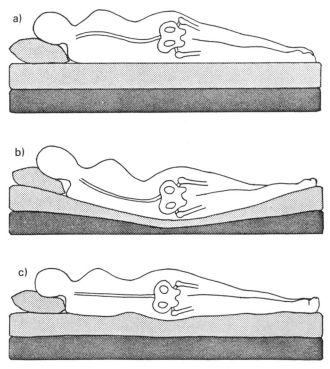

Figure 14 Mattress types: a) rigid mattress probably giving insufficient cushioning for shoulders and hips b) sagging mattress giving insufficient support for the spine c) ideal mattress giving both comfort and support.

Nowadays, the market is flooded with beds claiming to have been ergonomically designed by osteopaths or specialists in physical medicine. These are constructed from a variety of different materials and seem to have only one thing in common – they are expensive! An 'orthopaedic' bed may cost twice as much as a traditional bed and yet provide no extra comfort or support. Cost is immaterial as long as the bed provides the required degree of comfort and rigidity and is built to last. A simple mattress on the floor can be just as effective as the most expensive orthopaedic bed-set. My own preference is for a latex-foam mattress on a solid or slatted base. Other combinations are outlined in the table below.

GOOD BED GUIDE

Type of construction	Comments
Flock mattress on steel mesh springs.	Old fashioned and prone to sagging. Not recommended.
Interior sprung mattress on sprung base.	Generally too soft and liable to sagging. If used, select a firm edge in preference to a sprung edge.
Interior sprung mattress on solid base.	May give an acceptable degree of support, but choose pocket springing to avoid rapid deformation of the springs,
Foam mattress on sprung base.	The base generally makes this combination too soft.
Foam rubber on solid base.	Approaches the ideal in comfort and support
Foam mattress on wooden slats.	No improvement on solid base, but generally more expensive.
Water beds.	Provide adequate support if filled to correct pressure, but if too soft they make positional adjustments difficult. Costly.
Camp beds and hammocks.	Invite spinal strain and are best avoided, since they are rarely as comfortable as sleeping on the floor.

If you are currently sleeping on a traditional bed-set which seems excessively soft, make it firmer by placing a board under the mattress. Some people use an old door for this purpose, but it is better to employ a sheet of ¾ in (18 mm) blockboard cut specially to size. Alternatively, put the mattress on the floor and sleep on this, providing you will not attract the attention of passing cats, dogs, mice or draughts! Most hotels these days provide bed-boards on demand for back-sufferers. If they don't, and you find the bed you have been allocated too soft, ask to have the bed made up on the floor. Even if it is only for a single night, it is better to risk upsetting the management than risk upsetting your back.

But do not be surprised if your back is stiff and achy in the morning, even when you sleep on a bed of impeccable construction and design. Joints tend to grow stiff when they are idle, as they are for long periods during the night. As a result, if you have a back problem associated with joint or ligament stiffness, it is liable to be particularly troublesome in the morning after several hours of relative immobility. As a result, when you wake, you are likely to find it a struggle to get out of bed and bend to put on your socks and shoes – a condition some doctors refer to as post-inertial dyskinesia. Once you have had a chance to limber up, take a shower or make an early morning cup of tea, the stiffness goes and the back gradually becomes more comfortable. This period of early morning stiffness is one of considerable danger for back-pain sufferers. Many spines are strained in the first 15 minutes of the day by rolling out of bed, pulling on socks or tights or bending over a wash-hand basin. This risk can be minimised by observing the following early morning ritual:

☆ Before getting out of bed perform two simple exercises to stretch your spine. First lie on your back, clasp your hands round your knees and pull your knees firmly towards your chest. Repeat this movement six times, then stretch your legs straight out in front of you and push first your left foot and then your right as far as possible down the bed. Repeat this stretching movement six times with each leg; this will gently 'toggle' your pelvis from side to side and loosen the joints at the base of your spine.

☆ Develop a routine for getting out of bed which minimises the torsion at the base of your spine. Turn on your side with knees bent, as shown in Figure 15, then, in one smooth movement, drop your legs over the side of the bed so that you can use their weight to lever yourself into a sitting position, assisted by a gentle push from your elbows and hands. Do this while keeping the lower part of your spine as rigid as possible.

☆ Once on your feet, carry out some gentle movements to stretch your spine. Animals perform these loosening exercises instinctively the moment they wake to overcome their post-inertial dyskinesia. We should follow their example and ape the early-morning stretching movements of a cat.

☆ As far as possible, avoid heavy lifting and prolonged stooping during the first 15 minutes of each day. If you have to make your bed during this

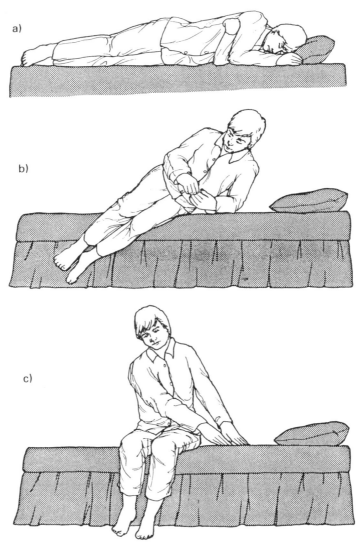

Figure 15 Getting out of bed: a) starting position b) keep the spine straight and use the weight of the legs to raise the trunk c) use a gentle push of the hands to get into a sitting position.

period, do so while kneeling on the floor rather than when bending from the waist. (If mattresses have to be turned, schedule this chore for midday on a Saturday, rather than first thing on a weekday when you are likely to be stiff, tense and pressed for time.)

Before leaving the subject of backs and beds, it is important to say something about the ideal sleeping position, if only to debunk some of the commonly held myths and old wives' fantasies. For years, people have struggled to avoid sleeping on their left side for fear that this would strain the heart. Others have endeavoured to lie on their stomachs throughout the entire night to improve their digestion, or face upward to protect their spines. Charles Dickens insisted on sleeping with his head facing due north to ensure the correct flow of the gravitational force through his body and, furthermore, carried a compass with him on his American tours to check that the furniture in his hotel bedroom was correctly aligned! People with varicose veins have been recommended to sleep with their legs higher than their chests and those with breathing difficulties to sleep with their chests higher than their legs. Enrico Caruso, the great Italian tenor, followed the advice of the day and slept propped up on a base of more than a dozen pillows, a practice which would have done nothing to improve his breathing and must have played havoc with his neck.

Many of these positions are exaggerated and unnatural and place considerable strain upon the spine. People who sleep face downwards are forced to twist their heads acutely to one or other side. This imparts a rotational strain on the spine which often injures the neck and can upset a sensitive lower back. Those who try to sleep on their backs throw their lumbar spines into a hollow, which can in time cause ligament strain. The safest policy is to fall asleep in whatever seems to be the most comfortable natural position. This will vary from individual to individual, depending on psychological factors as well as purely structural considerations, as psycho-analyst Alfred Adler pointed out as long ago as 1914. People who are insecure tend to protect their vulnerable parts by curling into a tight defensive ball. Those who are more relaxed and extroverted feel less need to guard themselves during the night and so adopt a more relaxed open pose. But these positions are of necessity open to frequent change. Providing you give the body a good base – a firm bed and a pillow of modest height – there is rarely any need to give conscious thought to the postural changes which the body will make automatically as and when it needs. The only exceptions to this rule are those rare cases when individuals have got into the habit of sleeping in a damaging position, perhaps with shoulders and legs turned to opposite sides of the bed, so that they twist the lower part of their back like a wrung-out dishcloth. Apart from these instances, which in my experience are very infrequent, it is safe to go on to automatic pilot during the night and let your sleeping positions be determined by a process of natural selection. Most of the time, you will probably end up in some variation of the side-lying, foetal position. This is the posture in which we were born and in which the Vikings, and no doubt many other races, were buried.

There is an ancient adage which says: 'The King sleeps on his back, the Wise man on his side, and the Rich man on his stomach'. Unfortunately I have had no opportunity to test the first clause of this proverb, and admit to grave doubts about the last, but I am in wholehearted agreement with the second. The side-lying position is generally a safe and comfortable posture for sleeping, as Figure 16 shows.

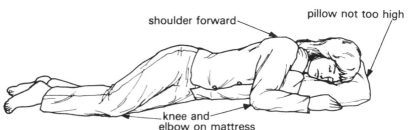

Figure 16 A comfortable sleeping position.

VERDICT The back can be injured by adverse sleeping positions and by strains incurred during the first few moments of the day, when the spinal tissues are liable to be at their stiffest. For this reason, it is advisable to use a bed of optimum resilience and practise some form of early-morning stretching exercises.

11 Foot Faults

It may seem incongruous to make mention of the feet in a book about bad backs and yet there is an exceedingly close link between the two areas. Twinges which start in the feet may all too readily end up as spasms in the back, or even as a pain in the neck!

This was appreciated by 'Old Bill', a shoe repairer whose wizardry with feet made his unpretentious cobbler's shop in London's East End a place of podiatric pilgrimage. Although Bill and I never met, I heard so many tributes to his artistry during my early days in practice that I came to trust his therapeutic skill. He would take patients with chronic backache and, after assessing the way they bore the weight on their feet, would subtly reshape the soles of their shoes, putting a wedge here and a supportive pad there. This would adjust their spinal mechanics enough to ease their postural strain. Other customers might come in complaining of tension headaches. A quick look at their stance, a glance at the bottom of their shoes to detect the tell-tale signs of shoe wear, then Bill would set about his task of constructing a shoe to correct their postural faults and ease their spinal strains. His success underlined the rationality of his approach. Both our stance and our gait depend on the way we balance our weight upon our feet. Introduce a slight torsion or tilt at the feet and the deviation will be carried on throughout the entire skeleton, often in magnified form. That is why back specialists need to be podiatrists as well as general physicians, ergonomists, psychiatrists and remedial gymnasts. As Dr Philip Lewin, Professor of Bone and Joint Surgery at Northwestern University Medical School, Illinois, wrote in the very first page of his excellent textbook *Backache and Sciatic Neuritis*: 'No back examination is complete without an examination of the bare feet, while standing'.

For the purposes of this book, there are four important considerations to bear in mind. The first is the question of heel height. I cannot remember how many times I have heard it said, often by supposed 'authorities', that high-heeled shoes are bad because they throw the weight of the body forward and so increase the arching of the back. This is a complete myth which, in the past, has led to all kinds of inappropriate therapy. A few years ago, there was a vogue for 'negative' heels, shoes which dispensed with conventional heels and substituted a raised platform under the forefoot so that the entire shoe sloped backwards from front to rear. The idea for these back-to-nature shoes came from Europe, but their merchandising and marketing mythology was 100 per cent American. The story proper starts on a beach in Denmark, for it was here that shopkeeper Anne Kalso noticed that, when people walk on sand, their heels sink lower than their toes. She decided that this must be the natural way to walk and, on this presumption, made some shoes with sloping soles which held the heels lower than the toes. She found these oddities comfortable to wear and introduced them as a novelty in her Copenhagen shop.

One of her early customers was Eleanor Jacobs, an American who was on a whirlwind tour of Europe with her husband. Eleanor's feet had grown tired of traipsing through art galleries and tramping over ancient monuments. The unaccustomed exercise had also given her an acute case of 'sightseer's back', which was marring the fun of her holiday. By the time she reached Denmark, she was in considerable pain and ready to try anything to relieve her suffering, even if it meant wearing shoes as inelegant as those in Anne Kalso's boutique. The new footwear proved an unexpected boon, easing the discomfort in her feet and relieving the pain in her spine. Thinking that they had found an answer to a major American catastrophe, the enterprising Jacobs bought the US patent for negative-heel shoes and, within a short while of returning home, had set up a production plant where they were soon turning out a million pairs of 'Earth Shoes' a year. Prospective purchasers were assured that wearing the shoes would help them stand straighter by lessening the hollows in their back. Unfortunately, none of the advertising copywriters bothered to check this claim, which was based on the assumption that, if high-heeled shoes throw the back into a hollow, as folklore insists they do, then shoes with a reversed tilt must have the opposite effect. But the claim is false for normally, when high heels are worn, the lumbar curve is flattened rather than increased.

This was proved by research work carried out, most appropriately, in the town where negative-heel shoes were first conceived. Three scientists attached to the Laboratory for Back Research, University Hospital, Copenhagen, studied the spinal curves of eighteen healthy women when they were wearing high-heeled shoes, when they were barefooted and also when they were wearing pairs of Anne Kalso's reverse-heel sandals. They proved that, when high heels were worn, the subjects maintained their balance by shifting their body weight backwards towards their ankle bones. This has the effect of flattening the lumbar curve. Conversely, when they wore the negative-heel sandals, they were forced to throw their weight forward to compensate for the backward tilt, which tended to increase the lumbar arch. In view of this, many doctors will have to revise their advice to patients with chronic back problems.

This, of course, is not the first time that medical opinion has been forced to make a therapeutic U-turn. Not so long ago, doctors were advocating low-residue diets for patients with colon disorders and the avoidance of all form of exertion for patients with coronary disease. Now the recommendation is a high-roughage diet for the colon-sufferers and a graduated regimen of physical exercise for the heart victims! As yet the news of the Copenhagen research has not filtered through to the majority of general practitioners. Until it does, readers of this book with painful, hollow backs should accept as proven fact that they may be more comfortable in high heels, especially when they are performing static tasks such as ironing, preparing vegetables, teaching or serving behind a shop counter.

High-heeled shoes, however, are not appropriate for active tasks like climbing stairs, negotiating greasy pathways or walking over uneven pavements. Nor are loose or ill-fitting shoes, shoes with worn heels, broken-down heel counters or excessively slippery soles. Many back injuries occur because people are improperly shod. The feet are the foundation stones of posture and the pivotal hinges of balance. In the summer, women may enjoy the airy elegance of sling-back sandals, but they do not provide the ideal footwear for clambering up the companion-way of a ship. One slip on a patch of uneven boarding and the spine may be thrown into a ligament-tearing contortion. In the ballroom, men may appreciate the smooth soles of their dancing pumps but these are not practical for everyday wear when they may be running up and down escalators and leaping on and off commuter trains. A recent survey at a British gearbox factory revealed that slipping was responsible for half the accidents which led to time off work. More detailed analysis showed that the low back was the most common site to be injured in these mishaps. This emphasizes the importance of slips and stumbles in the aetiology of back injuries. Anyone with a history of back trouble, or with a desire to protect their spines from avoidable damage, should wear shoes which give them a safe, solid footing on the ground.

Another precaution is to wear shoes which provide sufficient resilience to soak up some of the jolts and jars of daily life. During the course of an average day, our feet take a sledgehammer pounding of over 1,000 tons, some of which is transmitted to our backs. A certain amount of this impact is taken up by the feet, which are miracles of engineering ingenuity and, in an ideal state, make excellent natural shock-absorbers. The jarring would be infinitely worse if our feet were solid slabs of bone. As it is they each contain twenty-six bones, with seventy-two separate articular surfaces lashed together with ligaments and muscles to form thirty-three individual joints. This gives our feet the suppleness of a string of beads, the strength of a Roman arch and the resilience of a sprung seat. But even this is not enough to protect our spines from jarring when we walk and even more so when we run. In recent years, scientists have measured the shock waves which travel through the body when the heels strike the ground. They have discovered that, when we are walking on hard ground, our shins receive a jolt which is in the region of *five times* our body weight. When we break into a run, the force of these impacts soars to between ten and fifteen times body weight. Some of this jarring is absorbed by the knees and hips, but there is still enough left to give the base of the spine a sizeable thump with every step we take. Even the skull does not escape this regular pounding, getting a blow which, during running, is approximately equivalent to the total weight of the body. This explains why not-so-fit joggers sometimes suffer backache after running round the block and why people with hangovers tread so carefully when they step out of bed on the morning-after-the-night-before!

These jolts are minimised when we walk with economy of effort and smoothness of movement. But very few people walk well. Sit on a park bench and watch the world and his wife walk by and you will see how very badly they do it. You will see numerous hobblers, waddlers, mincers and strutters, but very few people who walk with elegance and ease. Those with a rigid or uneven gait are more liable to injure their backs. During walking, as each successive foot strikes the ground, the weight of the body should be taken first by the heel and then transferred in one smooth movement along the outside border of the foot and across the forefoot to the big toe, which acts as a launching pad giving a final lift and thrust as the foot leaves the ground. Excessive jarring occurs if the forepart of the foot strikes the ground first or if a flat-footed gait is assumed. The foot must be used like a rocking chair so that no one part of the foot carries the entire weight of the body for more than a fleeting moment.

People with back problems who find their pains are aggravated by walking over hard surfaces can lessen heel-strike jarring by wearing shoes with cushioned treads made of foam rubber or polyethylene foam. Yet greater protection can be gained by using heel pads or insoles made from Sorbothane®, which can be obtained from many major chemists and most sports-goods stores. This new, visco-elastic material has the ability to absorb 80–90 per cent of the impact energy of walking and provides an extremely useful foot-cushioning for runners, long-distance walkers and sufferers from foot, ankle, knee, hip and back disorders.

Back sufferers should take one final precaution: they should always make a point of walking with their knee caps facing directly forwards. This ensures the correct placing of the legs and allows the hinge joints of the ankle and knee to flex and extend easily, with no unnecessary rolling of the pelvis or unnatural twisting of the legs. This is a matter of considerable importance and is dealt with in greater detail in the chapter which follows.

VERDICT Wearing sensible shoes and walking with a smooth, natural gait can lessen the severity of chronic back pains. Since these measures improve general health and carry no risk of adverse side effects, they should be adopted by all back sufferers. Just 5 minutes' attention to the feet may save 5 months' treatment for the back.

12 Kipper Feet

Public relations consultants know the importance of proper timing. If they want to launch a new pop star, or unveil a revolutionary mouse trap, they do their best to choose a propitious moment when the attention of the media is not diverted elsewhere. They know that even the finest promotion can sink without trace if its advent coincides with a major press scoop, like a juicy political scandal or economic crisis. The same fate has befallen many important medical discoveries, which have received scant attention, not because they were of little intrinsic worth but because they were overshadowed by the course of subsequent events.

When World War 1 ended, doctors started to take a serious interest in patients with back problems. They were no longer content to believe that the rheumatic disorders stemmed from the circulation of an evil humour in the bloodstream, or from the absorption of poisons from the bowels. They felt there must be a mechanical explanation for many cases of lumbago and sciatica. An early product of this research was the identification of what came to be known as the Piriformis Syndrome. The first description of this entity, in a paper published in the *Lancet* in 1928, excited the medical profession, just as the world of natural history was roused a generation later by the discovery of the coelacanth, the prehistoric fish which had previously been thought to be extinct. Here was a possible cause of sciatic pain which was easy to comprehend and simple to cure. But, despite its attractions, the Piriformis Syndrome had a life span as brief as that of a mayfly. Before it had time to establish its place in medical practice, it was usurped by a charismatic upstart – the Slipped Disc. From the moment in 1934 when doctors were informed that bulging spinal discs could cause pain by pressing on the emerging roots of the spinal nerves, it was accepted that this was the only important cause of severe back pain and sciatica. All rival theories were forced into obscurity. As a result, most of today's medical students receive their degrees without hearing a single word about the Piriformis Syndrome, yet this remains a frequent cause of back and leg pain.

The condition gets its name from the piriformis muscle, a wedge-shaped muscle which arises from the inside of the pelvis close to the sacro-iliac joint; this muscle becomes progressively tapered as it runs outwards to finish as a tendon which is attached to the bump at the top of the hip bone. All anatomists agree that there is a very close relationship between this muscle and the sciatic nerve. In nine out of ten cases, the nerve runs under the belly of the muscle. In the remaining cases, the nerve takes one of three alternative routes. In just over 7 per cent of individuals, part of the nerve passes *through* the piriformis muscle; in slightly more than 2 per cent, part of the nerve loops *over* the muscle belly and, in nearly 1 per cent, the entire sciatic nerve travels through the substance of the piriformis muscle. In these anomalous situations in particular, it is possible for the sciatic nerve to become trapped or stretched by contraction of the piriformis muscle. This is the basis of the Piriformis Syndrome, which is characterised by pain in the buttock and leg which is often unrelated to movements of the spine, is usually not aggravated by coughing and sneezing, is relieved by rest and which is often most troublesome in the sitting position.

There are two reasons why the piriformis muscle is particularly prone to become bunched up and cause pressure on the sciatic nerve. In the first instance, the muscle derives some of its attachments from the ligaments spanning the sacro-iliac joint. Any strain of this joint can therefore cause reflex protective spasm of the piriformis muscle. The second reason for the peculiar vulnerability of the piriformis muscle is less easy to explain, but of considerably greater significance. When we stand or walk, we bear a large part of our body weight on our heel bones. These are slightly offset, the point of contact the bone makes with the ground being always *outside* the body's weight mass. This means that there is a natural tendency for the heels to roll inwards whenever we assume the erect position, a movement which is normally checked by the pull of the muscles which maintain the inner arches of the feet. If we grow lazy or tired these muscles relax and our arches flatten and the inner borders of our feet roll inwards. This rolling movement, or pronation, is always associated with an inward rotation of the shin bone because of the oblique angle of the main foot joint (subtalar joint).

This movement can be detected even by a layman. Sit down, take off your shoes and place your feet firmly against the ground. Now feel the knobs on either side of your ankle joint. You will notice that the bony bulge on the inside of your ankle (internal malleolus) is placed slightly further forward than the bump on the outside (external malleolus). Now obliterate your arch by rolling your feet inward. You will find this can only be done by twisting the entire shin bone, so that the internal malleolus is rotated backwards almost in line with its partner on the outside of the foot. This is what happens whenever people walk with a flat-footed gait. This tends to rotate the whole leg inwards. As it is awkward and ungainly to walk with the knees pointing inwards, the body steps in at this point and makes an automatic adjustment. It rotates the entire leg outwards from the hip joint. This still leaves the feet in a badly pronated position, but corrects the alignment of the knees so that they are in the right plane to carry out their simple hinge-like movements during walking. This is the best the body can do to correct the faulty gait, but the compensation has one serious mechanical drawback.

The piriformis muscle is an external rotator of the hip joint and will become shorter and fatter whenever the leg is held in a position of outward rotation. This increases the risk of sciatic-nerve compression. If the leg is held permanently in this position, as happens whenever people walk with flat, kipper feet, the muscle undergoes adaptive shortening. This makes it less elastic and therefore more prone to strain. An awkward twist getting out of a two-door car or a stumble on a loose paving stone and one or other piriformis muscle may be strained. This causes the muscle to become painfully cramped and swollen, a state which may put tension on the sciatic nerve. This happens not infrequently. When it does, it is useless to apply treatment to the back, whether it be by manipulation, injections, diathermy or spinal supports. All such attempts are doomed to failure from the start, yet they are often persevered with for months in the mistaken belief that *all* back and leg pains emanate from the spine.

There is one simple way to detect if the piriformis muscle on one side is shortened or in spasm. Lie relaxed on the floor for a few moments thinking about the weather, your mother-in-law, the state of your bank balance or anything but the placing of your legs. Then glance down as the position of your feet. If one naturally and habitually drops out further than the other, there is a probability that the piriformis muscle on that side will be either shortened or contracted (see Figure 17). Now raise each leg in turn about 9 in (23 cm) from the ground and try and swing it across its partner. This movement is limited in cases of piriformis shortening and can be excruciatingly painful in the Piriformis

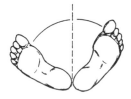

Figure 17 Shortening of the piriformis muscle causing outward rotation of the leg.

Syndrome, when the contracted muscle is putting tension on the sciatic nerve. (Tests on corpses show that raising a straight leg puts tension on the piriformis muscle long before it stretches the sciatic nerve.) Strangely enough you are more likely to find piriformis shortening on the right-hand side of your body than on the left. This coincides with the finding that outward rotation of the leg is more than twice as common on the right-hand side than on the left. This may be due to an asymmetry of weight bearing, for it has also been noted that five out of six children have a right foot which is broader than the left. A further test of piriformis shortening is to lie on the back with hands clasped around the knees, as shown in Figure 18. In this position, each knee in turn should be rotated inwards. Since we rarely perform this movement, it often becomes restricted and, when attempted, produces a sharp, catching pain in the groin. But if the movement is noticeably more limited or painful on one side than the other, it is likely that the piriformis muscle on that side is shortened. This *may* be the cause of pain radiating from the buttock down the back of the thigh and along the outer aspect of the shin.

Immediate relief for piriformis pain can sometimes be obtained by lying on a bed and getting a willing helper to apply a firm downward pull on the ankles. A more effective way of relieving spasm in the piriformis muscle is to carry out the rotational movement shown in Figure 18. This should be performed slowly and *gently* several times a day for periods of not more than 2 minutes at a time.

The yoga exercise known as The Twist is another effective way of stretching the piriformis muscle. If the trouble has its origins in faulty body mechanics, as is so often the case, an attempt must be made to improve the gait and foot placement. Correct the trend to walk with the legs turned outward like a penguin and check the tendency for the feet to roll inwards by wearing shoes with a strong inside counter and by strengthening the arch-supporting muscles. This can be done quite simply after taking a bath or shower by balancing on one leg while lifting

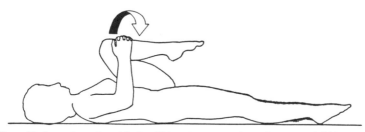

Figure 18 *Inward rotation of the leg. This movement can be used as a test of piriformis shortening and also as a corrective exercise.*

and drying the other. For obvious reasons I call this the Stork exercise. Where the pronation of the feet is more difficult to correct it may be helpful to wear specially-made orthoptic applicances in the shoes.

VERDICT *This is a generally neglected cause of sciatic pain, which can often be speedily relieved by appropriate treatment. Contractions frequently develop in the piriformis muscle. When these are found they should be corrected even when they are not giving rise to immediate pain, since they interfere with free-ranging leg movements and predispose to back strain. Restoring the normal elasticity of the muscle can do nothing but good, unless the stretching exercises are performed with excessive zeal, in which case they will be counter-productive, causing additional pain and further protective muscle spasm.*

13 Movement Is Life

If you gather together a score of orthopaedic surgeons, physical medicine specialists, osteopaths and rheumatologists, and ask them to describe the medical treatment of chronic back pain, you can be sure of getting at least twenty different replies. The regimens suggested will vary enormously, with just one notable exception. They will all include a schedule of back exercises. Specialists know from experience that spines benefit from being used. The well-exercised back has greater suppleness to prevent injury, greater strength to resist strain, greater stamina to stave off fatigue and better co-ordination to maintain balance. Regular movement also helps to work off the muscular tensions that build up round the spine and improve the circulation so that minor injuries are more easily healed.

Tests show that back pain is more common in people with weak muscles and stiff joints. In one trial, a group of subjects were given a simple flexibility test. They were asked to bend down and try to touch their toes with knees straight. If they couldn't make both ends meet, a measurement was taken of the gap between their fingers and toes. The test revealed that back pain was more likely to persist or recur the greater the loss of spinal flexibility. This is why elderly people so easily damage themselves in stumbles and falls. The consequences of falling down a flight of stairs varies from person to person and from age to age. When babies fall down stairs, they bound like rubber balls. Such is their suppleness that, when they reach the bottom of the flight, they are probably suffering no more than bruises and shock. Not so the elderly or stiff. They only have to trip over a single tread to suffer an acute back strain or hip fracture. And it is not only senior citizens who are at risk. Even youngsters are peculiarly susceptible to back injuries if they are abnormally stiff.

When doctors examined a group of nearly 500 schoolchildren attending a comprehensive school in Norwich, they found that a quarter had back pain, generally at the base of their spine. For a third of the youngsters, aged between 13–17 years, the trouble was bad enough to warrant a visit to a doctor, to stop playing games or to take time off school Further investigation showed that this high rate of juvenile invalidism was more commonly found in youngsters who were stiff than in those who were supple, and in those who were not games players than in those who took a reasonable amount of physical exercise.

Backache is one of the hypokinetic diseases, one of the wide range of contemporary disorders linked with lack of exercise. The yogis have a saying: 'Movement is life'. This is particularly true of the health of the back. Our spines need movement for five main reasons:

☆ To maintain the strength of the supporting muscles which cushion the spinal joints from strain.

☆ To provide relief from prolonged postural strain.

☆ To relax muscular tensions.

☆ To retain the suppleness of the spinal joints.

☆ To uphold the strength of the bony skeleton. This is a vital, but little known, function of general exercise. Many elderly people develop postural stoops because their bones become soft and fragile, sometimes through nutritional deficiencies but more commonly as a result of disuse atrophy. Laboratory experiments show that subjecting the hind legs of rabbits to pressure increases the density of their vertebrae. This is the sort of stimulus that human beings get quite naturally when they walk or run. The more we use our spinal muscles, the more we encourage the circulation to our spines and the stronger our vertebrae and spinal discs become. Researchers at the postgraduate medical school, Hammersmith, London, have proved this in post-mortem studies on human corpses. These reveal that the mineral weight of the vertebrae is directly proportional to the weight of the muscles spanning the front of the spine. In fact, the more we use our bodies, the tougher our bony framework becomes.

For many years, spinal exercise programmes have been directed toward the development of muscle strength. In my experience this emphasis has been misplaced. With our sedentary life styles, we don't need bulging muscles. We are unlikely to be asked to dig canals or carry hundredweight sacks of cement. The most energetic tasks we are likely to tackle are digging the garden and playing a game of squash and, providing we start these jobs gently and perform them regularly, we will almost certainly develop the muscle strength we need to carry them out in safety. What we more commonly lack today is suppleness. This is particularly true of people who are under stress or who perform largely sedentary work. They need to carry out daily exercises to maintain the suppleness of their spines. This is as true for teenagers as it is for the elderly.

As the years go by, our connective tissues lose some of their original

68

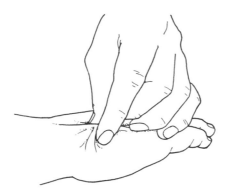

Figure 19 Pinch test to show flexibility of the connective tissues.

flexibility. This is easily demonstrated by taking the pinch test (see Figure 19). Lift a fold of skin away from the back of your hand, then release it and see how quickly it springs back into place. When you are young, the skin flattens out almost immediately. At 50 years old, the ridge of skin remains visible for about 2 seconds; at 70 years, it lasts sometimes as long as 30 seconds or more. Similar changes take place in the spinal ligaments and intervertebral discs. As parents and grandparents, we lose some of our spring when we step down from a chair and find it not quite so easy to bend down in the morning to put on our socks and tie up our shoes. Some of this loss of flexibility is inevitable, but a lot more is self induced. Nature makes us stiffen, but it is idleness that makes us painfully stiff. I have examined people who have carried out spinal stretching exercises throughout their lives and who, as a result, were able to bend down and touch their toes in their 90s. Over the years, I followed the progress of a famous ex-dancer who kept up her morning workouts at the barre long after she retired, with the result that she was still high-kicking in her late 80s. At 60 years old, film star Gracie Fields continued to defy her age by going on stage and turning cartwheels and doing the splits and, at the age of 65 years, birth-control pioneer Marie Stopes could still perform her party trick of putting her big toe in her mouth. By carrying out regular stretching exercises, these agile oldies were able to retain much of their youthful suppleness and spring.

Hatha yoga is one of the finest systems of exercise for the spine, particularly if it is combined with natural strengthening activities, such as walking, swimming, dancing and tennis. These age-old movements and poses are gentle enough for people of all ages and levels of physical fitness and are ideal for improving posture, encouraging relaxation and maintaining flexibility. A number of my patients have overcome their recurrent back problems by taking up yoga. Some, when I have had the

69

opportunity to examine them after a lapse of time, have been more supple at 70 than they were at 50 years.

A short while ago the Yoga Biomedical Trust carried out a survey of 3,000 yoga enthusiasts, to determine why they had taken an interest in this ancient Hindu cult of physical culture and what benefits they had derived. More than a third mentioned backache as one of their reasons for taking up yoga. Of these, 98 per cent reported that regular practice of the yoga had helped to ease their spinal pains.

A short while ago, the directors of the Owens-Illinois Glass Company, the world's largest glass manufacturers, grew alarmed at the high incidence of sickness absenteeism among their employees caused by back problems. On the advice of a specialist in physical medicine, they instigated an exercise programme for their staff. Foremen were trained to spot the tell-tale signs of lumbago and sciatica. The moment workers showed the slightest sign of stiffness when they straightened up from their work benches they were invited to step back from the production line and perform a standardized set of exercises to loosen their spines. If this failed to bring relief, they were sent to the factory clinic where a specially trained physiotherapist loosened their backs with manipulation and assisted stretching exercises. This simple regime of treatment brought quick returns. Within 15 months, the firm's toll of absenteeism from low-back troubles had fallen to a tenth of its previous level. Not surprisingly the directors of the company declared themselves 'astounded and gratified' by the results obtained.

There are many schedules of back-rehabilitation exercise. Some are more effective than others and a number positively dangerous. The ones I favour were devised nearly 50 years ago by Paul C. Williams, a consultant orthopaedic surgeon attached to the Parkland Memorial Hospital, Dallas. They are designed to improve the flexibility of the back and to correct the common tendency to over-extend the lumbar spine. They exclude backward-bending exercises simply because these movements often aggravate back troubles. Many spines are excessively hollow to begin with, so do not want to be further arched. Extension of the lumbar spine also places additional strain on the vertebral joints, raises the pressure within the intervertebral discs by 140 per cent and increases the risk of spinal-nerve compression. For these reasons, painful spines should not be subjected to excessive backward bending. In the words of Professor Williams: 'There is no justification for ever including in a low-back program the exercise that consists of lying prone and arching the back'. Yet in most hospitals this is the exercise that forms the basis of most back-rehabilitation programmes. It is given for the best of reasons but frequently has the worst of consequences. Tests carried out some years ago at Guy's Hospital, London, revealed that half the back-pain patients attending the hospital's outpatients clinic were made worse by performing the usual routine of back-extension exercises.

The exercises which follow are both simple and safe. They should be carried out slowly and deliberately at least once a day. If any movements cause pain, they should be stopped immediately and not resumed until expert advice has been obtained. Carrying out these exercises regularly will secure a marked improvement in spinal flexibility within a month. This is no idle promise; this has been proved by trials carried out at the University of Texas Health Science Center, Dallas. In this study, a comparison was made between the range of lumbar movement of two groups of people of comparable age. The first group had back pain, the second had done. Measurements showed that the patients complaining of pain were invariably stiffer than their partners who were pain-free. On average, the patients could manage no more than 37° of lumbar movement, whereas the controls could swing their lumbar spines through an arc of 82°. To overcome this handicap, the patients were instructed to perform the Williams' exercises three times a day. At the end of 3 weeks their range of movement was once more tested. This time they showed an average range of 65° of lumbar movement, a remarkable increase in spinal flexibility of 72 per cent!

THE WILLIAMS' EXERCISES

Exercise 1 is designed to strengthen the abdominal muscles. Adopt the position shown in Figure 20.1, then raise the trunk as far as possible and try to place the folded arms on the knees. Repeat 5–20 times depending on age and physical condition. People with stiff spines or weak abdominal muscles may be unable to do this exercise unless they fix their feet under a suitable piece of furniture.

Exercise 2 follows naturally from the preceding exercise and is designed to strengthen the gluteus maximus, the large buttock muscle which plays a major part in supporting the trunk in a forward flexed position and in preventing excessive hollowing of the back. Bring the feet to within about 9 in (23 cm) of the buttocks and place the hands on the abdomen just above the navel to make sure that the lumbar spine is not lifted from the ground. Now contract the buttock muscles so that the pelvis is rotated backwards. This will have the effect of rolling the pelvis so that the tail is lifted and the base of the spine pressed firmly against the ground. Repeat 10–20 times.

Exercise 3 is my favourite movement for back-pain sufferers, since it does all manner of helpful things in a way which is invariably safe and soothing. Its main effect is to obliterate the lumbar curve, relax tense muscles and stretch out chronically stiff ligaments and joints. Place the hands around the knees and pull them as close as possible towards the chest. Repeat 10 times. The best effect is obtained from this exercise when the head is kept relaxed on the ground and when only the very base of the spine is lifted from the ground.

Exercise 4 is also designed to improve the flexion of the lumbar spine but has the added effect of stretching any contraction of the hamstring muscles. As it also imparts a strong pull on the sciatic nerve, it should not be performed by people who are experiencing pain radiating down their legs. Start from the sitting position and bend the trunk forward

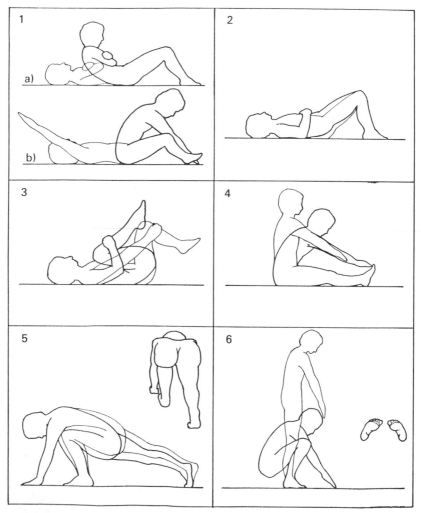

Figure 20 The Williams' exercise schedule. 1 Strengthening the abdominal muscles: a) basic exercise b) less strenuous version. 2 Strengthening the buttocks. 3 Obliterating the lumbar curve. 4 Improving flexion of spine and loosening the hamstrings. 5 Stretching the tissues on the front part of the pelvis. 6 The native squat.

trying to touch the toes and bring the head as close as possible to the knees. Relax and repeat 10 times.

Exercise 5 is designed to relieve stiffness in the connective tissues spanning the front of the pelvis which limit extension of the hip (mainly the iliofemoral ligament and the fascia lata). Adopt the position shown in Figure 20.5, with the left leg bent and the right extended straight behind you. Keep the left foot planted flat on the ground, then bend the left knee and press the pelvis towards the ground so that a definite stretch is imparted to the front of the right thigh. Carry out 10 stretches of the right hip then change the position of the legs and repeat the movement on the opposite side.

Exercise 6 is another favourite of mine which I call 'the native squat'. It serves a number of functions, including flexing the lumbar spine, stretching the heel cords and strengthening the thigh muscles which play an important role in postural control. Stand with feet about 12 in (30 cm) apart and toes turning outwards. Then bend the trunk and sink into a deep squat, keeping the heels firmly planted on the ground. Hold this position for a short while then resume the standing position. This is the position which peoples of the Third World countries maintain for hours on end, but which many Westerners find difficult to adopt, particularly if they are used to wearing high-heeled shoes. Ideally, the exercise should be performed in bare feet, but shoes with low heels may be worn to begin with if it is initially impossible to perform the exercise with heels flat on the ground. Later, as the heel cords stretch, the shoes can be discharged.

This exercise should not be performed by people with knee problems such as arthritis or cartilage damage.

VERDICT: Exercises play a vital part in the relief of chronic back pain and in the prevention of back injuries; but they must be chosen with care and they must not be performed if they give rise to added discomfort.

14 Making Light Work Of It

Some occupations carry a high risk of back injury. In industry, the traditionally vulnerable spines have been those of dockers, foundry workers and miners. A study of the causes of sickness absenteeism among these three groups of heavy manual workers shows that back trouble is responsible for 68, 66 and 63 per cent of their total invalidism. These figures have probably dropped somewhat since this survey was taken, due to the increased mechanisation of their particular industries. Other jobs are less easily automated, like nursing, which is particularly prone to cause back strain. A survey in Finland showed that nine out of ten nurses had suffered at least one episode of back pain, the risk being particularly great for nursing aides, who on average did twice as much heavy lifting, bending and twisting as qualified nurses.

The close relationship between back pain and repeated manual handling strains at work has been clearly demonstrated in an investigation carried out by Professor Peter Davis and his team from the Department of Human Biology at the University of Surrey. The researchers were invited to study the incidence of back injuries among various categories of Post Office workers in the UK. The men were classified according to the strenuousness of their work, using a radio pill to record variations in their intra-abdominal pressure, a measurement which is known to be closely related to the strain imposed upon the spine. When the results of the survey were analysed it was found that heavy manual workers, who regularly carried out tasks which pushed their intra-abdominal pressure up to 100 mm/Hg, had nine times as many episodes of back trouble as light workers, who rarely, if ever, achieved such high pressures. The activity which was found to impose the highest strain on the back was lifting an object from the ground with legs straight, particularly if the trunk was slightly twisted at the time. Facing the load, keeping the legs bent and lifting the weight from a raised platform all helped to ease the strain on the spine.

The evidence clearly shows that physical stresses and strains at work are a common cause of back trouble. This toll of sickness, invalidism and suffering could be substantially reduced if the following commonsense

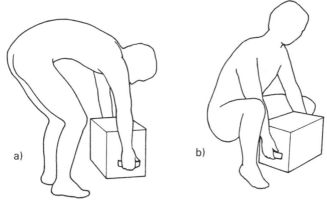

Figure 21 Lifting techniques: a) incorrect method b) correct method, standing close to the load with the spine straight and the feet firmly balanced.

measures were introduced:

☆ *Lifting techniques*   Everyone should learn how to lift, not when they take their place on the job market, but in their first few lessons in the school gymnasium. The skill is easily mastered and, once acquired, soon becomes a matter of habit (See Figure 21). The instructions are these:
a) Stand as close as possible in front of the load with the feet placed about 18 in apart, one foot being behind the load, the other slightly to one side. This provides a firm base and reduces the risk of stumbling.
b) Now sink into a crouched position, keeping the knees bent and the spine straight and get a firm grip on the object.
c) Lift with the arms straight and load held as close as possible to your body, by using the powerful muscles of the leg. This removes all risk of spinal strain.

Load Limits Currently Under Consideration In The UK.

Weight	Recommendation
Under 35 lb (16 kg)	Can be safely handled by all but those with special limitations, providing proper lifting techniques are used.
35–75 lb (16–34 kg)	Workers regularly lifting weights of this magnitude should be screened to eliminate those with back problems.
75–120 lb (34–55 kg)	The regular manual handling of these weights should be confined to workers who are trained and properly supervised; otherwise mechanical hoists should be used.
Over 120 lb (55 kg)	At this level, manual handling systems should be employed whenever possible. When this is not practical, the work should be restricted to those few people who are strong enough to perform the task with safety.

☆ *Load limits* When it comes to lifting heavy loads two pair of hands are invariably better than one. Don't overestimate your strength and don't be too proud to ask for help. Over the years various welfare bodies have issued safety limits for manual lifting.

Women should take particular care when lifting, since their muscles are generally weaker than those of men and their manual handling capacities on average are 30 per cent less. Even athletic girls should take care when bending to handle loads, since the configuration of the female pelvis sets the centre of gravity of the body behind the axis of the hip joints, which creates a mechanical disadvantage when lifting in the stooped position.

☆ *Lift and shout* Pupils of the oriental martial arts are trained to give a bloodcurdling scream when they aim a karate kick. Infantrymen are taught to do the same when they make a bayonet thrust. Others make their explosive efforts with a less ferocious shout. Jimmy Connors became famous for the grunt he gave with every smash serve, and the sport of competitive weight-lifting would hardly be the same without the varied groans and cries uttered as hefty barbells are hoisted overhead. Making these cries appears to make lifting easier, according to research work carried out in Ohio, USA. In these trials, it was found that the lifting ability of students and soldiers increased by an average of 15 per cent when weights were raised with an audible cry. Even greater gains in strength were recorded by women who employed the lift-and-shout technique.

Scientists are not too sure why the method works, but believe that there is normally a mental block that prevents us from exerting our full force. Giving a loud shout, they think, helps us to overcome our inhibitions and to focus our entire animal force on the task in hand.

☆ *Pulling and pushing* Jobs requiring regular pulling movements are likely to strain the back, but much less so than work involving repeated pushing. This was revealed in a study of over 300 workers carried out by scientists from the University of Vermont. They divided the workers into three groups: those who experienced no back pain, those who had moderate backache and those who suffered severe pain. They then determined how many pushing units they registered each day, the score being obtained by multiplying the weight of the object moved by the number of times it was shifted. The results showed that the workers with no pain averaged 326 pushing units a day, those with moderate pain 532 units, and those with severe pain 1,612 units. A similar, but lesser, correlation was discovered between back pain and repeated pulling.

Why should pushing be so dangerous for the spine? The answer to that question has been provided by Professor Peter Davis and Dr D.A.

Stubbs of the University of Surrey. They used the standard technique of feeding volunteers with a radio pill to measure the build-up of pressure within their abdomens. This gave them a continuous report of the strains their spines experienced. With this aid, it was revealed that subjects could *pull* with a force of 80 lb (36 kg) without putting any appreciable strain on their backs. But if they used the same force to *push* a load, the tension levels soared to danger limits. In view of this, if there is a choice, weights should be dragged rather than shoved, using the weight of the body to do as much as possible of the work. Loaded wheelbarrows should be pulled up steps rather than pushed, with the arms held straight and the main lift coming from the extension of the thighs. The same principles apply to manhandling an immobilised car. Here it is generally difficult to get a decent grip on the front of the car, but the body doesn't mind if the pulling is done from behind. This may sound an impossible proposition but, as far as the muscles of the back and thighs are concerned, the strain is the same whether a car is being pulled from in front with the hands or pushed from behind with the back. Imagine yourself pulling a car by means of a rope lashed around its front bumper; then visualise yourself in the same position and, at the same time, leaning backwards against the rear of another car, which you are attempting to shift by the backward thrust of your shoulders and back. By leaning back and forcibly straightening your legs, you can either pull the car in front of you or shove the car behind. In either case, the effort and dynamics are the same. By using one or other of these techniques, cars can be moved with far less risk of back strain than when using the more popular forward thrust.

☆ *Load-carrying* To minimise strain on the back, weights should be carried as close as possible to the spine. A short while ago, two Indian researchers carried out a series of experiments to discover the simplest, safest way of carrying heavy loads. They took seven volunteers and set them the task of carrying 70 lb (38 kg) of granite chips in a variety of different ways. Sometimes the stones were carried in the hand, at other times on the head or in a back pack. The results revealed that the strain was reduced when the load was symmetrically balanced and carried as close as possible to the spine. The least efficient method was to carry the weights in the hand. The technique involving least strain was the unusual double-pack harness, a device developed for use by commandos during World War 2 (see Figure 22). In the Third World, people are generally much more efficient at carrying weights than Westerners. They carry loads on their heads rather than in hand-held suitcases, shopping baskets and briefcases. Their babies are strapped to their backs or perched on their hips, whereas we carry them in our arms or in cumbersome carrycots. Worse still, we often burden ourselves down every day with

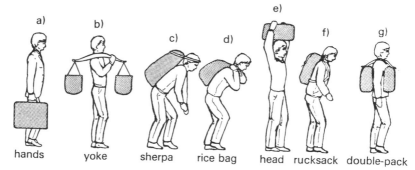

Figure 22 Load carrying. Seven versions ranging from the least efficient (a) to the most efficient (g).

unnecessary paraphernalia, carrying handbags stuffed with papers, keys and miscellaneous bric-a-brac and attaché cases loaded with files, magazines and electronic gadgetry. We would do well to tip out our personal holdalls every week and strip them of their surplus bits and pieces. The same applies to the briefcases and dufflebags carried by youngsters going to and from school. A team of Austrian doctors, led by Professor Karl Chiari of the Vienna University Orthopaedic Clinic, grew alarmed at the frequency with which children developed spinal curvatures. When they started school, five out of six children had a straight spine; when they left, more than one in two had developed a spinal deformity. The curvatures, the doctors thought, might be caused by carrying heavy loads of books. So they took a sample of the children and weighed the contents of their school bags. The results were alarming. On average the children were regularly carrying a weight of 24 lb (11 kg), the equivalent of carrying six railway carriages in one hand in a single school year. To lessen this strain, the team recommended the use of loose-leaf textbooks, which can be taken home a page or two at a time, and a return to the old-fashioned satchel which was worn on the back rather than carried in the hand.

Anything which lightens the loads we carry lessens the risk of back strain.

☆ *Bending and stooping* Jobs which involve regular stooping, like housework, dentistry, nursing and paper-filing, carry a high risk of back trouble. Researchers have measured the amount of bending involved in these jobs with some startling results. They have developed a 'flexion analyser', a battery-operated instrument which straps on the back and records all bending and straightening movements. With its assistance, they have discovered that dentists spend about 52 minutes per hour in a semi-fixed position. During this time, they, perform an average of eight additional stooping movements. But their work is light, since the only load they carry when they bend and straighten is the weight of their own trunk. Nursing aides suffer more back strain because their work is heavier. When they flex their spines, they may be making beds, picking up slop pans or lifting patients. They spend about half their working time in a flexed position and, during the course of an hour, make an average of seventy deep forward flexions. Warehouse workers spend slightly less time in the flexed position (just over 27 minutes per hour) but made over 150 deep bends per hour when they are often lifting heavy loads. These are revealing findings, which suggest that the toll of back pain in industry could be reduced by restructuring jobs to lessen the need for bending and stooping. This can often be done by the introduction of appropriate machinery and the correct placing of work surfaces. Housewives would suffer less back trouble if their ironing boards and kitchen tops were at a suitable height. Ideally, to eliminate stooping, they should be able to brush their knuckles on work surfaces when they stand erect. Eye-level cookers, raised cupboards and the shoulder-height placing of commonly used kitchen utensils can all help to reduce excessive bending and stretching in the kitchen.

A lot of the stooping we do in the course of the day can be avoided. A team of American ergonomists used a flexion analyser to study the work patterns of a group of janitors both before and after they had attended a back-care training programme. The results showed that, once the men had had the prophylactic training, they reduced by half the number of deep forward bends they made. As a further benefit, it was found that they spent a third less time in a back-straining, semi-flexed position.

☆ *Accidents* Injudicious lifting, pulling, stooping and carrying are not the only cause of on-the-job back strains. Many injuries occur through accidental stumbles and falls. When the Health Education Unit of a South London borough carried out a survey of back-pain sufferers, it was found that only one in seven attributed their back injuries to a lifting strain, whereas over 50 per cent thought their strains had resulted from an accident at work, an accident in a car, a fall, an illness or playing a sport. Accidents at work can be avoided by clearing passages of likely stumbling blocks and mopping up oil spills. In the home, the common causes of accidents are over-polished floors, loose or worn mats, climbing insecure ladders, standing on rickety chairs to remove curtains or replace broken light bulbs, insobriety, poorly lit landings and staircases and stumbles over hazards placed on staircases and hallways. (The details of these accidents were fed into a computer, which noted that a high proportion of falls occurred on the bottom or top tread of staircases; so it printed out as its major recommendation for accident prevention: 'Remove top and bottom step from all staircases'.)

VERDICT Hard work kills nobody, but can give rise to crippling back pains. These work-related pains can be substantially reduced by taking sensible precautions when lifting, load handling and carrying. Steps should also be taken to avoid needless bending and stooping.

15 Getting Knotted

Most people are familiar with the concept of psychosomatic disease. If they were asked to provide a list of the most common tension disorders, they would probably mention peptic ulcers, high blood pressure, colitis, migraine and heart attacks; but would possibly overlook back pain. Yet many cases of lumbago and sciatica are stress-related. London taxi drivers are under constant tension with their work. Some suffer nervous indigestion, all too many have heart attacks and a number end up on my treatment couch complaining of stiff necks and tense, aching backs. One of these patients claims to be the most placid cabbie in London because he has found that, if he loses his temper at the wheel, he quickly notices shooting pain travelling down his leg. The threat of this stabbing pain is enough to make him keep his cool however much he is provoked!

We appreciate that our facial muscles are organs of emotional expression which accurately mirror our mood when we are happy, angry, sad or afraid, but we do not generally recognize that the same applies to our spinal muscles. Yet we notice the mood-linked postural changes in the spines of four-footed animals. The family Dalmatian will bow his head in shame if he is caught with his head in the refrigerator, showing a typical hang-dog look, while the neighbour's cat will arch her spine and hiss defiantly if the Dalmatian leaps the garden fence and pays her an unwelcome social call. Similar changes occur in human beings. It is not difficult to differentiate the members of two sporting teams when they quit the field after a keenly contested match. Both have laboured equally hard and yet their postures are totally different as they make their way to the dressing room. The victors hold their heads erect and walk tall; the vanquished slump dejectedly. Elation is always associated with an upright carriage of the spine; failure and dejection with a drooping posture. Fear is accompanied by an increase in tension in all the postural muscles, which is seen most readily in animals which freeze rigid when they are confronted by a powerful adversary. The same can happen to us if we are attacked at night by a mugger. Fear throws us into a straightjacket of muscular tension and, though we long to take some purposeful action, we can neither raise a scream nor lift an arm in self defence. A similar response sometimes grips fledgling soldiers when they are first plunged into action. This occurs, according to ancient Norse legend, because Odin strikes his adversaries with an invisible bolt which causes a paralysis called 'battle-fetter'.

Although we may not always be aware of these tension changes in our spine, we do acknowledge them in our conversation. Some of our most colourful expressions of emotional response describe these innate postural changes. When someone annoys us, we say 'they get our backs up'. When we are frightened, we claim to be 'scared stiff'. People who grieve are 'bowed down with sorrow'; those who are beset with troubles suffer so much tension in their upper backs that they sometimes feel as if they 'were carrying the load of the world upon their shoulders'. Others irritate us to the extent that they become 'a pain in the neck', or more vulgarly 'a pain in the arse'.

Nowadays it is possible to measure these changes of tension in the paraspinal muscles by a process known as electromyography. Some years ago two British physicians, Drs Peter Sainsbury and T.G. Gibson carried out some revealing experiments with this equipment, which records the changes of tension within a muscle by measuring the minute variations in electrical activity. They put patients complaining of tension pain through a deliberately stress-provoking interview. When they placed their recording electrodes on normal muscle tissue, they noted a slight increase in tension during the interview, which quickly diminished the moment the experiment was over. But when they placed the electrodes on muscles which were normally the site of tension pain, they observed a totally different response. The reaction then was exaggerated, with the troubled muscles continuing to contract, even when the interview was over, and remaining tense for some while afterwards.

People who suffer tension back pains tend to be over-reactors, who put their backs into everything they do. Sometimes this causes tension headaches, sometimes fibrositis in the shoulders and, at other times, low backache or sciatica. Everyone tends to have their own target site. In practice, I have found that people with anxious or aggressive personalities are more likely to suffer from stiff necks and tension headaches, while depressed or lonely people are more prone to experience tension pains in their legs and lower back. This general impression has been supported by experimental work carried out recently by Dr Walter Oosterhuis at the University of Amsterdam. He studied the psychological status of 500 patients who were complaining of pain for which there was no obvious physical cause. Some were overly aggressive, some fearful, others in a state of obvious despair. Investigation showed that the psychological state determined not only the onset of the pain but also its precise location. Of the many patients who expressed feelings of aggression, over

97 per cent complained of pain in their neck. Of those who experienced fear, 90 per cent suffered pain in the abdomen: while 60 per cent of those in a state of despair felt pain in their lower back. Lumbago can sometimes be the sign of a drooping psyche rather than a slumping spine. I have found it to be common in lonely people, as did Dr Iain Gilchrist, a Manchester doctor who investigated 1,500 of his patients and found that low backache was twice as common among divorced and separated people as among those still living with a spouse.

In the past, the medical profession has been somewhat unkind to patients suffering from psychosomatic back pains. Some have been accused of being hysterical, others of malingering. In cases where the pain resulted from an industrial accident, for which insurance disability payments could be obtained, a diagnosis of 'compensationitis' was sometimes made. In the USA this was occasionally referred to as the 'green poultice syndrome', since it was thought to respond miraculously to the application of $100 bills. In 30 years of practice, I can only remember one person whom I considered to be suffering from a truly hysterical back-pain syndrome and only a handful who were trying to take financial advantage of their suffering. In my experience, people may exaggerate, elaborate or prolong their symptoms, but they do not invent them. Back pain is rarely, if ever, purely *imaginary*.

Some people, of course, find that their bad backs provide them with a socially acceptable excuse for not digging the garden or making love to their wives. Others use their symptoms as a cry for help. A wife may have a husband who is so wrapped up in his work that he treats her with neglect, except when she has a bout of lumbago, when he suddenly becomes a loving, attentive companion. This may encourage her to magnify her disability in order to get the attention she craves. Others yearn for sympathy, sometimes as a substitute for a genuine, intimate loving relationship with which they cannot cope. They will invariably dramatise their symptoms to capture the pity of anyone who cares to give them an audience, painting vivid pictures of nerves torn to shreds and daggers thrusting into their back. Phlegmatic patients generally give an accurate assessment of their disability and will admit that their pain is limited to certain areas of the body and is relieved by changes in position or certain treatment measures. On the other hand, sufferers seeking a pay-off reward will tug at the heartstrings of their listeners by telling of agonising pain which spreads from head to toe and never lets up for a solitary moment. These people need both physical treatment and psychological support.

A patient's posture is important in determining his or her likely response to treatment, and this refers as much to their mental posture as to their physical stance. To recover from back pain, it is not only important to find the right therapist but also to have the right mental attitude. This applies whatever the treatment, whether it is surgery, drugs, bed rest, exercises or manipulation. Three American doctors proved this when they investigated a series of back-pain patients attending a single orthopaedic clinic. All were given a preliminary structural examination and a detailed psychological investigation before they were treated either by surgery, bed rest or epidural injections. Subsequent analysis showed that the psychological examination was a more accurate predictor of their response to treatment than the medical examination, blood tests, X-rays and electromyograms. Depressed patients showed a particularly poor response to treatment, irrespective of the surgeon's initial assessment of the severity of their physical condition. When treating back pains, it is as important to know what sort of person has the pain as to know what sort of pain the person has. Yet many doctors find it far easier to cope with mechanical disturbances than to handle emotional ills. Their training equips them to repair broken legs but not to mend a fractured ego. Many grow impatient when depressed individuals hold on to their aches and pains, despite receiving the finest drug treatment or the most skilled manipulative therapy.

In the years ahead, we may expect tension to play an increasingly important role in the aetiology of spinal pain. Atavistic physiological changes occur within our bodies whenever we are under stress. These are necessary for our self defence. When primitive man came face to face with a sabre-toothed tiger, his muscles tensed, his pulse raced and his blood pressure soared. This prepared his body for fight or flight. Whatever course of action he chose, the stressful situation was quickly relieved. Either he raced away to the safety of his cave, clubbed the beast to death or died in the struggle. Not so with the stress we experience today. A man may spend a lifetime at loggerheads with his boss which makes his hackles rise. After their first clash, he feels the muscles in his back tense but he resists the temptation to pick the fellow up and throw him out of the office window. Instead he retains the tension in his trunk muscles and this gradually builds up to produce genuine pain. Others suffer because they have been trained to bottle up their emotions. As children they were taught to conceal all show of feeling. 'Brave boys don't cry'. 'Nice girls don't make a scene'. 'Pull yourself together'. 'Don't wear your heart on your sleeve'. 'Keep a poker face'. All these familiar admonitions train us to become more and more tense. We are afraid to let ourselves go in case we let the mask slip. Wilhelm Reich, at one time Freud's favourite pupil, showed how people control their emotions by holding themselves in a straightjacket of muscular tension. They erect what he described as a 'body armouring' which prevents them feeling pain. They tense their diaphragms to hold back the tears and contract their pelvic and abdominal muscles to still the rumbles of fear. Some of this protective tension is found in the back and several times I have relaxed a patient's back only to release a torrent of tears. By freeing the body armouring, I had released the flood gates of emotional expression.

Tension is also aroused because we live in an age of high anxiety. Every time we switch on the television or open the paper, we receive reports of brutal murders, street violence, famines, rapes and civil wars. In response to this stressful bombardment, we become anxious and tense. Like a flock of birds or a herd of cattle, we respond immediately to the distress calls of our fellows. But, unlike these animals, our response is purely passive. We hear the alarm call but we do not react to it by taking any form of physical action. We don't take flight from the happenings that alarm us, or fight the entity that makes us afraid. So tension persists and may make itself felt as a stiff neck or aching back.

Noise also plays a part in creating tension. Just before the start of World War 2, Landis and Hunt, two American scientists, published a book called *The Startle Pattern*. This described research into the atavistic response of both men and animals to the sudden noise of a gun fired at close range. They recorded the startle response with high-speed ciné-cameras capable of taking as many as 3,000 frames per second. These sequences were then played back at normal speeds so that the bodily reactions could be observed. They showed that, although the startle response starts with an involuntary blinking of the eyes, it quickly spreads downwards to involve the rest of the body. Within half a second the neck is thrust forward, the shoulders hunched, the abdomen contracted and the trunk arched. The only difference noted in the reaction of the human guinea pigs and their mammalian counterparts was that the human beings did not prick up their ears when they heard the blast. Otherwise we tense up in exactly the same way as a rabbit or monkey every time we hear an unexpected noise – a door slam, a telephone bell, a police siren, a low flying jet or a backfiring car. Since these nerve-shattering blasts are a regular accompaniment of city living, our backs are constantly suffering the convulsive jerks of the startle response.

In time our muscles become adapted to being held in a state of constant contraction, whether the tension is caused by noise, body armouring or repressed emotion. Eventually the muscle fibres actually shorten, as German physiological research has shown. This represents a saving of energy, but causes a loss of flexibility which makes the tissues more prone to strain. This creates a vicious circle in which tension leads to stiffness and pain, and stiffness and pain to further tension and added pain. In the end it is difficult to tell which came first, the chicken or the egg, whether the disorder is psychosomatic in origin or somatopsychic. In the same way it is frequently impossible to determine whether a patient has back pain because they are depressed or whether they are depressed because they are in constant pain. Often there is no point in trying to make the theoretical distinction.

What is certain is that, in cases of chronic back pain, benefit can often be obtained by relaxing the tense spinal muscles. This can be done on a purely palliative level by taking a hot bath or having a thorough body massage. More permanent relief can be gained by adopting a more relaxed life style, learning to avoid needless anxiety and non-productive worry, lowering ridiculously high goals and standards and endeavouring to be less fussy about trivial issues.

But the finest way of overcoming tension in the back is to take some form of physical activity. When we react to emotional stimulation, our spinal muscles contract as a preparation for some kind of physical activity. We suffer pain only when this activity is repressed, when for some reason we choose to have the emotion without the motion. There are times when it would be anti-social to act as our instincts dictate, when we don't want to throw a temper tantrum or punch our neighbour on the nose. On these occasions, it is useful to work off our tensions in other ways. Animals do this quite naturally. They are rarely the victims of passive stress. When they are afraid, they run. When they are annoyed, they bellow with rage. If they are trapped or frustrated, they struggle to set themselves free. And, on those rare occasions when they do not directly lift the lid off the emotional pressure cooker, they will find some alternative way of giving vent to their pent-up tension. Ethologists refer to this behaviour as displacement activity. Instead of fighting, antelopes will dissipate their anger by clashing their antlers against a tree, herring gulls will tug at tufts of grass and stickleback fish will stand on their heads and dig holes in the sand with their snouts. By engaging in these harmless rituals, they quickly and safely dispel their tension states.

People suffering chronic tension pains in their back can benefit by indulging in similar displacement activities. They can sublimate their accumulated tensions by digging the garden, felling trees or playing squash. Better still, they should take part regularly in rhythmical exercises like swimming, cross-country walking or free-style dancing. These are the finest antidotes for victims suffering from the effects of a stressful, sedentary life style.

VERDICT *Tension is a contributory factor in many chronic back-pain syndromes. It can be relieved by learning to relax, by adopting a less stressful life style and by indulging in regular, rhythmical exercise.*

16 Whited Sepulchres

Long before we had X-rays to detect the presence of vertebral decay and blood tests to spot the build-up of uric acid or alkaline phosphates, doctors took a very simplistic view of the rheumatic diseases. They did not bother to differentiate between Paget's disease, gout, ankylosing spondylitis and disc prolapses. As far as they were concerned, every ache or pain in a muscle or joint was due to the build-up within the body of an evil humour called 'rheum'. When this exuded from people's eyes, they were said to be rheumy-eyed. When it settled in their backs, they were diagnosed as suffering from rheumatism. The treatment for these excesses was to rid the body of its store of accumulated toxins, a cleansing that was done by blood-letting and purging, measures of universal application which were often infinitely more distasteful than the maladies themselves.

This theory could not be upheld in an era of scientific medicine but it was such a useful explanation for all the conglomeration of rheumatic aches and pains that it could not be discarded altogether. Just as pagan customs did not disappear completely with the arrival of Christianity, but became subtly transmuted into respectable Christian feasts, like Christmas and Easter, so many primitive healing cults have been transmogrified and perpetuated in more acceptable form by giving them a veneer of scientific respectability. This happened with the humoral theory of rheumatic disease which was tailored to meet the more exacting requirements of scientific scrutiny at the start of the twentieth century.

In 1920, it was suggested that most cases of lumbago, sciatica and fibrositis resulted, not from the distribution of a mythical noxious humour, but from the spread of toxins from hidden pockets of infection within the body. This theory of 'auto-intoxication' proved highly acceptable to a medical profession which had only just been weaned from its centuries-old dependence on the humoral theory of disease, and was equally attractive to laymen brought up on the doctrine of original sin. They were quite happy to believe that physical sickness was due to a poisoning of the flesh, just as they had been led to accept that evil thoughts and deeds were the root cause of the mental suffering of individuals and the moral decay of nations. Like whited sepulchres, our glistening outer shells hid festering sores. 'We must turn our attention inwards', the health educators of the day proclaimed, 'and rid our bodies of these breeding grounds of disease'.

While this hunt was on, countless healthy teeth were drilled, kidneys flushed, bowels purged, sinuses irrigated and tonsils and appendices removed in an endeavour to rid the body of hidden foci of infection. Some of the most influential doctors of the period were engaged in this mass crusade of ritual purification. Notable among them was Sir William Arbuthnot Lane, an eminent surgeon from Guy's Hospital who was convinced that the absorption of toxins from the lower bowel caused not only rheumatism but also tuberculosis, heart disease, high blood pressure and insanity. To cure these myriad ills, he recommended a healthy diet, abdominal belts and copious doses of liquid paraffin. If the patient was adequately fit and sufficiently wealthy, he took the more radical step of excising their colons, an operation he performed more than a thousand times. Other doctors were content to give their patients rheumatic pills which contained either diuretic drugs to flush their kidneys or aperients to wash out their bowels. In either case, the aim was to achieve a state of inner cleanliness, an attractive slogan adopted by more than one laxative manufacturer.

When further research showed that many cases of low-back and sciatic pain resulted directly from mechanical defects – prolapsed discs, bony anomalies, vertebral degeneration – the auto-intoxication theory was declared a heresy. Now it is rare to hear it mentioned by any self-respecting doctor, and rarer still to find it detailed in any textbook of rheumatology. This is regrettable because, in my mind, there is no doubt that infections can aggravate rheumatic pain. Anyone who has had a bout of influenza and suffered stiffness and aching in every muscle and joint will not need convincing of this fact. In my experience, localised infections remote from the spine are rarely if ever a primary cause of back pain, but they can aggravate or bring to light existing troubles. This is also the opinion of Dr Paul C. Williams who, for two decades, presented an Instruction Course at the American Academy of Orthopaedic Surgeons. 'I believe that a focal infection is capable of initiating clinical symptoms in dormant mechanical lesions, making it impossible to obtain relief by mechanical measures until the infection is over', wrote Dr Williams when describing the causes of low-back pain. He listed the sinuses, adenoids, teeth, gall bladder, urinary tract and prostate as common sites of focal infection.

Infection can also spread from gum disease, a disorder which affects most adults in the civilised world, according to the World Health Organization. In a state of health, the teeth are surrounded by a tight

88

collar of gum tissue which ends in a tight, sharp fringe rather like the cuticle at the base of a finger nail. This gingival fringe seals the tooth and prevents food debris and bacteria from entering the tooth socket. If the gums are allowed to become diseased, they become soft, swollen and tender instead of hard and firm. This weakens the seal around the tooth and permits the formation of small pockets in the gums where food debris can lodge and bacteria multiply. This leads to a condition known as pyorrhoea, which literally means a 'flow of pus'. Some of this infected material can be absorbed into the circulation and carried to traumatised tissues in the back, where it can irritate pain-sensitive nerve endings. This possibility was emphasized by a speaker at a recent dental congress: 'The bacteria and toxins from gum infection may be absorbed into the bloodstream and even the gastro-intestinal tract, where they are thought to be a significant contributory factor in a wide variety of diseases'. The rot may start in the mouth, or gall bladder or sinuses, but it does not necessarily stop there. So if you have any reason to believe that you might be suffering from any form of chronic infection seek appropriate medical help from your doctor, dentist or gynaecologist. Don't be a martyr to persistent infection which might be sapping your vitality and aggravating your rheumatic pain.

VERDICT *Chronic infections of the sinuses, teeth, gall bladder and female genital organs can never be a cause of acute back pains and sciatica, but they can exacerbate chronic backache. Removing these sources of infection is always advisable, for, even if it does little to ameliorate your spinal pain, it will at least improve your general health.*

17 Going For A Stretch

From the cradle to the grave we are engaged in a ceaseless struggle to defy the forces of gravity. The battle begins in infancy, when, as toddlers, we rise unsteadily to our feet and take our first faltering steps, and it continues throughout life until we finally give up the unequal struggle and lay ourselves down to die. In between these times, our tissues are dragged down by the inexorable gravitational pull which makes our arches fall, our wombs prolapse, our bellies sag and our breasts droop. The spine is subjected to the same deforming force. It is as if we were constantly carrying a heavy weight upon our heads, which, as the years proceed, compresses our discs and increases the bowing of our spines. Most people who suffer back trouble long to be relieved of this concertina force. 'I'd love to be fixed in a rack by my feet and hands and pulled in opposite directions', is the plea I often hear. This is an understandable reaction, for stretching the vertebral column does reverse some of the adverse effects of gravity and can help to correct structural deformities and relieve spinal pain. Some of my patients have invented the most ingenious ways of stretching their spines. One leading artist devised an ankle harness connected to a block-and-tackle so he could hang upside down from the ceiling whenever his back grew tired at the end of a day's painting.

This is the basis of one of the oldest recorded treatments for spinal disorders. Two thousand years ago, Hippocrates, the father of modern medicine, published a treatise on *Fractures, Joints and Instruments of Reduction*. This described a primitive method of spinal traction in which patients were tied by their ankles to the bottom-most rung of a ladder. The ladder was then grasped on either side by two sturdy assistants and tipped upside down, so that the sufferers were suspended by their feet. This reversed the effect of gravity and imparted a strong pull to the spine, which separated the vertebrae and eased the pressure on any compressed spinal nerves. If tougher measures were indicated, the ladder was raised a foot or more in the air and then allowed to drop to the ground so that the spine received an additional, corrective jerk. Nowadays, traction is applied in hospital in a somewhat more controlled fashion, with the patient lying in bed with a harness fastened about the waist attached to weights dangling from a pulley fixed at the end of the bed. The *modus vivendi* has changed but the effect remains the same.

Four-footed animals rarely suffer back pain. They owe their immunity in large part to the fact that they hold their trunks in the plane that nature intended. The intervertebral discs make excellent shock absorbers when the spine is in a horizontal position but they were quite obviously never designed to carry prolonged vertical loading. Like the hydraulic buffers at the end of railway lines, the discs are charged with fluid which makes them excellent structures for soaking up intermittent jerks and jolts but they do not take kindly to constant compression, which squeezes out some of their fluid content, making them flatter and less pliable. This long-continued compression may also interfere with the normal nutrition of the discs, making them more prone to degenerative change. The body contains arteries which run for an estimated 60,000 miles (nearly 10,000 km). They carry vital nourishment to the innermost recesses of the muscles, heart, kidneys, lungs and brains but they do not penetrate the spinal discs. Discs have to be fed in a totally different way. Microscopic examination shows that the layers of cartilage which separate a disc from the vertebrae above and below are perforated by a network of tiny holes like slices of aerated bread enveloping a cheese sandwich. This permits an interchange of fluid between the vertebrae and the intervening discs. When the pressure in the discs is high, fluid is forced into the vertebrae; when the pressure falls, fluid is sucked back into the discs. This explains why we lose height as the day proceeds, fluid being slowly squeezed out of the spine's twenty-three discs, making each one that much thinner than when the day began. Although the individual difference is small, the overall effect is sufficient to make us lose ½–¾ in (0.6–1.9 cm) in height during the course of the day. When we go to bed the pressure in the discs falls by about 86 per cent. This permits the rehydration of the discs and allows us to regain our full height during the course of the night's repose.

Some years ago, I was approached by a police inspector who wanted help for a young cadet. The boy had proved a promising pupil but unfortunately was just short of the minimum height requirement to join the regular force. 'Could you suggest any treatment to help the lad grow?', the inspector asked. As the youngster's posture was good, he could not add to his stature by standing more erect. So I gave what, in the circumstances, was the only possible practical advice. 'Keep the boy in bed until the very moment he has to take his medical', I suggested. 'Then see that his height is measured before any other tests are taken'. Although I received no official report, I understand that this simple ruse worked and the boy achieved the necessary height qualification. Had he failed to make the grade, I would have needed to recommend sterner measures, like sending him in orbit round the moon! This greatly reduces the pressure on the discs and leads to more marked increases in height. This explains why astronauts gain anything up to 1 in (2.5 cm) in height when they travel in space and are subjected to conditions of zero gravity.

Just as spines grow when the pressure on them is relaxed, so they tend to shrink when the pressure on them is increased. Tests at Nottingham University show that carrying a 30-lb (14-kg) load on the shoulders doubles the rate of disc shrinkage. This leads to bulging of the ring of fibres marking the perimeter of the disc (annulus fibrosus), which heightens the risk of nerve compression. Scientists have found a yet more ingenious way of shrinking the spinal discs. They noted that pilots testing ejector seats suffer a loss of height when their torsos absorb the sudden shock of being propelled from the cockpit of their planes. Furnished with this evidence, they then carried out measurements on circus artists taking part in the Human Cannon Ball act, and discovered that they too lost height, generally in the region of ⅜ in (0.95 cm) when they were blasted through the air.

So far there are no reports of astronauts getting miraculous relief of back pain when they float through outer space but there is a modest amount of evidence that these pains can be eased by self-applied traction, which stretches the spine and can relieve the pressure on the spinal nerves. Tests show that a traction force of 60 lb (30 kg) reduces the pressure within the discs by about a quarter.

Ten years ago, Harriet Barber suffered what she described as 'an acute and horrendous backache'. Her family doctor despatched her to the local hospital where she was treated with bed rest, traction and 4-hourly shots of morphine. Within 10 days she had recovered sufficiently to be sent home but an injudicious sneeze brought the pain back in all its old intensity, so she was rushed back to hospital for further treatment. Over the next 2 months, she was shunted backward and forward between her home and the orthopaedic ward, her pain and disability getting gradually worse. Eventually she was admitted to one of Nevada's premier orthopaedic hospitals, the Washoe Medical Center in Reno. Here specialists put her through a battery of tests, took a myelogram of her spine and diagnosed that she was suffering from a ruptured disc which would most probably require surgical treatment. But her husband had other ideas. He had heard that back pain could be cured by hanging people upside down by their feet and had decided that this ancient cure deserved a trial before his wife submitted herself to the surgeon's knife. So he set to work at the family ranch to construct a tilting table from bits of rubber tubing, scrap plywood and lengths of discarded steel pipe.

Eventually his Heath Robinson device was completed and he faced his major challenge. As Harriet later recalled: 'His most difficult accomplishment was talking me into coming home from the hospital to try his bit of nonsense'. It was her husband's enthusiasm that finally won the day and, soon after making the painful journey home, Harriet found herself being helped into the makeshift device, which the family quickly nicknamed the Back Rack. Her feet were secured in rubber loops and the platform gradually tilted backwards until she was hanging at an angle of about 45°. 'As I went backwards, I immediately had freedom of back pain', she relates. 'I couldn't believe it; this monstrous piece of junk really worked!'

It would be nice to report that Harriet is now completely cured but in truth she is still prone to a recurrence of severe pain if she neglects her homework for too long. If she takes a daily stretch on the rack, however, she keeps free of pain without the need for analgesic drugs, and she finds this simple precaution infinitely preferable to making regular hospital visits or undergoing disc surgery. As for her husband, he was so pleased with the success of his invention that he refined it, patented it and re-christened it the 'Backswing', a name his friends found a little less awesome than the original Back Rack. This device is now marketed throughout the world, where it has found favour with countless members of the Bad Back Club.

Another inversion device was developed by Dr Robert Martin, a Californian orthopaedic surgeon. He constructed a range of anti-gravity boots which clip on to the feet rather like ski-boots. These contain a projection behind the ankle which can be hooked round an overhead bar, so that back-pain sufferers can take the pressure off their spines by hanging upside down from their toes, like bats. Dr Martin does not claim that this is a panacea for all back problems, although he can now point to thousands of satisfied users who regularly look at the world through topsy-turvey eyeballs.

The manufacturers of these devices are careful to warn potential customers of their possible side effects. Since inversion therapy became popular in the early 1960s, there have been reports that the treatment can provoke congestive heart failure, uncontrolled hypertension, hiatus hernia and haemorrhages in and around the eyes. In a study at the Chicago College of Osteopathic Medicine, a group of healthy medical students were examined while hanging upside down from anti-gravity boots. In all cases it was found that, after 3 minutes in the inverted position, there was a significant increase in pulse rate, blood pressure and intra-ocular pressure. This led the researchers to warn that inversion therapy should be used with caution, especially by those suffering from high blood pressure, heart disease or eye troubles.

Some doctors find it preferable to avoid these hazards by stretching the spine in the erect position. This is a technique which Newmarket family doctor, Dr A.E. Dossetor, has been using in his practice for many years. He has a conveniently placed cold-water pipe running across the top of his surgery door and, some while ago, he decided to use this to try to straighten the backs of patients who came to him in the familiar corkscrew position. While he wrote out a prescription for a pain-killing drug or muscle-relaxant tablet, he got them to hang from the pipe. His aim was to widen the space between the vertebrae and so ease the pressure on the spinal nerves. While they were suspended in this position, he asked the patients to raise their knees and swing them gently from side to side. If necessary he applied a gentle shove to aid the rotary movement. Sometimes the patients 'felt a click' in their backs, an event he welcomed since it often signalled a dramatic lessening of their pain and muscle spasm. After he had manipulated 2,000 backs in this way, he published an enthusiastic report in the *British Medical Journal*. Only a few of the patients he had treated needed to be absent from work for more than a week, many being able to return to their work-places straightaway. As a result, he told colleagues, 'I would like to recommend this technique for the treatment of backache'.

This is a remedy that can readily be given at home. Horizontal bars can easily be fitted in the framework of a door, and these will serve the same purpose as Dr Dossetor's water pipe. A simple alternative is to drape a folded towel over the top of any convenient door. This gives a comfortable hand grip from which back-pain victims can hang for as long as they can bear. In this position, the knees should be gradually bent and the pressure slowly lifted from the feet so that the spine is stretched by the downward pull of the legs. Keep the trunk as relaxed as possible and hold the stretch for 1 or 2 minutes, then slowly straighten the knees so that the weight is once more taken by the feet. Make these movements as smooth as possible, so that the spine is not subjected to sudden, painful jerks, and repeat the complete cycle of traction and release one or two times until the hands tire. Added benefit can sometimes be gained by rocking the pelvis backwards and forwards while the spine is being stretched, but none of these movements should be performed if they cause pain. If you try this technique, make sure you observe two simple precautions. In the first place, the door should be wedged in the open position so that there is no risk of it swinging shut and trapping your fingers! Secondly, take care to apply your weight as close as possible to the hinges, so you do not prise the door from the wall. Providing you observe these safeguards, the only risks you run from hanging from a door, trapeze, overhead beam, horizontal bar or chandelier are strained shoulder muscles and blistered palms.

VERDICT *Although traction is still a favoured hospital treatment for bad backs, it has not come out well in clinical trials, several of which show that it has no noticeable effect on pain, spinal mobility or neurological symptoms and signs. Although it undoubtedly produces a lowering of pressure within the spinal discs, the reduction recorded is only a third of that which occurs when lying down, a procedure which is simpler, cheaper and generally much more comfortable! Strangely enough, the greatest benefit of traction seems to be enjoyed by elderly patients with chronically stiff backs which show X-ray evidence of degenerative change. Short spells of hanging may benefit these patients, accompanied by gentle mobilising movements of the trunk when there are mechanical problems, such as locked facets or fragmented discs. If inversion therapy is attempted, the tilted-frame method should be chosen in preference to the anti-gravity boots, since the angle of hang can be graded according to individual needs and levels of tolerance. In this case, follow the manufacturers' instructions, starting the treatment gently and only gradually increasing the angle of inclination and duration of stretch. Before you invest in any of these devices, give them a thorough pre-purchase trial for some people are particularly sensitive to being up-ended and, in that position, suffer an unacceptable level of nausea, dizziness or head pain. Seek your doctor's advice if you have any doubts about the safety of these methods and never hang upside down if you suffer from high blood pressure, heart disease, recent strokes, 'drop attacks', glaucoma, conjunctivitis or retinal detachment.*

18 Rest A While

Rest is a universal panacea. The overworked businessman on the verge of a nervous breakdown takes a 3-months' vacation from his job. The teenager who goes down with glandular fever retires to bed. The patient recovering from a major operation is sent away to a nursing home to convalesce. In these situations, relieved of unnecessary stress and strain, the body is enabled to make full use of its innate powers of recuperation. Rest and time are the great healers but, like all other powerful remedies, they are not without their untoward side effects.

At one time, a badly sprained ankle would be immobilised in plaster for 6 weeks. Then it was discovered that this led to adhesion formation and the development of a joint which was unnecessarily stiff and weak, so the strapping was made lighter and the length of immobilisation shortened. This did not depress the sale of plaster of Paris, however, for, as soon as it was deemed unwise to overprotect a sprained ankle, it became therapeutically fashionable to encase injured backs in wrap-round plaster jackets for anything from 2 to 6 months. Eventually this idea was also discarded, when it was realized that prolonged immobilisation stiffened the spinal joints and weakened the back muscles. Now it is mainly neck injuries which are treated by immobilisation, cervical collars being the in-vogue orthopaedic appliances at present – one wonders how long it will be before they too are used with greater caution.

Complete bed rest may seem the sanest and safest option for recent back injuries and yet no two specialists seem agreed on when or how it should be applied. If a patient with sciatica goes to hospital X, he may be put to bed for 4 weeks and not even allowed up to visit the toilet. If the same patient, with exactly the same symptoms, chances to go to hospital Y a few miles away, he may be enrolled immediately for a course of strenuous physiotherapy exercises. I have even known patients who, on visiting an orthopaedic clinic, have been offered the choice of bed rest or exercises! If the specialist cannot decide between these diametrically opposed therapies, it seems unreasonable to place the burden of selection on the layman. How can the choice be made?

Bed rest helps the damaged spine in three main ways. In the first place, it relieves the pressure on the spinal discs. When a man weighing 11 stone (70 kg) stands erect, the pressure within his lumbar discs rises to approximately 22 stone (142 kg). When he lies down in bed, the pressure immediately drops sevenfold, to roughly 3 stone (20 kg). This reduction in intradiscal pressure can be beneficial when pain is being caused by the pressure of a bulging disc on a spinal nerve. Bed rest also relaxes the postural muscles of the back and pelvis, which again can relieve pressure on trapped spinal nerves, but, more important than either of these two factors, it lessens the irritation of inflamed tissues. If a nerve is trapped by a bulging disc, arthritic outcrops or distorted spinal joints, it becomes swollen and inflamed. This causes pain and an increase in muscle tension, which, in all probability, further aggravates the pressure on the nerve. A nerve nipped in this way needs to be rested rather than tweaked from side to side by repeated movements of the trunk and legs. It is rather as if one's ear lobe was being gripped in a pair of pincers. The vice-like hold itself would be painful enough, without added tugs and twists of the pincers. The same applies when back pain emanates from a spinal joint. The excessive use of a recently sprained spinal joint is damaging because it increases pain and swelling in the joint, just as it does with an injured ankle or wrist.

On the debit side, bed rest carries three main risks. In the first place, enforced idleness leads to rapid muscle-wasting, which makes the back weaker and more prone to subsequent strain. It also hampers the circulation, which slows down the healing of damaged tissues and retards the drainage of areas of congestion. Equally important, immobility favours the formation of restrictive scar tissue. Whenever a muscle, joint or ligament is injured, there is an immediate flow of blood into the damaged tissues. This leads to the formation of a blood clot, which contains a mesh of protein fibres (called fibrin) together with thousands of fibroblasts, the cells responsible for the formation of new fibrous tissue. Within 24 hours of the initial injury, a dense network of fibrous tissue is laid down to repair the wound, in a pattern which is totally dependent on the mechanical forces prevailing at the time. If damaged ligaments or muscles are gently used as they heal, the repair tissue is laid down along the line of longitudinal tension, as Nature intended but if they are kept slack the fibrous tissue is deposited in a totally haphazard fashion, with the result that bridges may form between ligaments and bones or between adjacent muscle fibres. This undesirable binding can be a cause of subsequent pain and restricted movement. The same thing can happen to joints which are allowed to stagnate after an injury. In this case, adhesions form within the joint and can become a cause of persistent pain and restricted movement.

When a back is acutely injured, the ideal is obviously to gain all the benefits of bed rest while incurring none of the attendant penalties. This is more easily achieved than might at first be thought. The secret is to adhere to two simple principles:

☆ When a back is injured, it should be subjected to as much gentle and frequent movement as it can stand. This will maintain muscle tone, improve the circulation, reduce swelling, hasten the repair of damaged tissues and prevent adhesion formation. Naturally, this advice does not apply to people who have been involved in major car accidents or in falls from sixth-floor windows and who might have sustained a spinal fracture, but it is applicable to the vast majority of back injuries. Spines were made to be moved and are better able to cope with the problems of use than with the less obvious hazards of inactivity.

☆ Any movement which aggravates pain should be avoided. Pain is an excellent yardstick for people recovering from back injuries. Some are in agony the moment they stand on their feet or walk more than a few yards. They should heed Nature's warning and spend as little time as possible in the erect position. Others are happy standing or walking about but are in agony the moment they sit down. They should keep on the move as much as possible and, if necessary, eat their meals off the mantelpiece. I have known people who could not sit in comfort at an office desk for more than 10 minutes but who could play a vigorous game of squash without noticing the merest twinge. They were not work-shy malingerers for, in each case, there was an excellent anatomical reason for them being happier on the move than sitting down. They were safe to carry on playing squash but were strongly advised to give chairs a wide berth until their pain abated. No two cases of acute lumbago are quite alike and so the prescription of exercise and rest can never be exactly standardised. What suits one person may just as easily aggravate another. Nevertheless, over the years, I have proved the universality and safety of the instruction 'Exercise gently and frequently within the limits of pain'. Even when patients are unable to move from their beds in comfort, I advise them to take some form of gentle exercise, such as the gentle knee-hugging described on page 71, the pedal-pushing movement outlined on page 53 or the deep breathing mentioned on page 143. This I am sure eases pain, hastens recovery and limits the risk of adhesion formation.

The cautionary remarks which apply to bed rest apply with even greater force to the wearing of restrictive spinal corsets. These cumbersome devices have most of the drawbacks of prolonged recumbency with few compensatory advantages. Wearing a corset, for instance, does not reduce the pressure within the spinal discs, nor does it fully protect trapped spinal nerves from irritating tugs. But it does limit injudicious bending and, by providing a tight binding round the waist, it does increase the pressure within the abdomen and so gives added support to the spine. As it happens, both of these functions can be achieved by other, simpler means. Forward bending can easily be limited by applying two or three strips of non-stretch adhesive strapping along the back from shoulder blades to buttocks. This was a favourite remedy in my student days, when patients with acute spinal problems would be manipulated and then returned to work with their backs protected by a few strips of 2-in (5-cm) wide adhesive plaster. I remember distinctly the smell of the tincture of benzoin we applied to the skin beforehand and recall even more vividly the painful task of removing the plaster casing when its task was done. But I believe the remedy served a useful purpose, if only as a temporary warning not to stoop or twist.

The other main function of the spinal corset, the support of the stomach wall, can be performed equally well by an old-fashioned abdominal belt. The Victorian manual worker – gardener, docker or farm labourer – always girded his waist with a hefty leather belt. This was not to hold up his trousers, since he invariably wore braces for this purpose. Nor was it to provide protection for the sacro-iliac joints, as some have suggested, for the belt was normally worn around the waist rather than circling the pelvis. The only conceivable reason for wearing thick, tight belts around the waist is to raise the pressure within the abdomen and so increase the hydraulic support for the spine when heavy weights were lifted. The modern competitive weightlifter invariably takes advantage of this aid, gaining support by wearing a thick leather belt around his waist. A spinal corset will undoubtedly have the same effect, but is unnecessarily restrictive to other movements and also cumbersome to wear.

Corsets, like bed rest, should be used sparingly. They can provide a measure of support in the first few days of an acute back injury, just as a plaster cast protects a broken limb, but they should be discarded after 6 weeks unless a specialist advances a specific reason for continuing their use.

VERDICT *Bed rest and spinal corsets are not universal panaceas for acute back injuries. Both have their contra-indications and should be used sparingly. The safest policy after a back strain is to exercise gently and frequently within the limits of pain. As a prophylactic measure, manual workers involved in heavy lifting may find it useful to wear a supportive abdominal belt.*

19 Blowing Hot And Cold

For centuries, sufferers from fibrositis, lumbago and sciatica have found relief by wallowing in hot water. Generations of Japanese have eased their aches and pains in communal bath houses. In Ancient Rome, as many as 3,000 people at a time soaked away their tensions and twinges in the gigantic public baths. In Georgian England, those who could afford it took their rheumatic joints to fashionable spas, such as Cheltenham, Bath and Tunbridge Wells, and, in France, famous society hostesses like the 50-year-old Madame de Sévigné went to Vichy to follow a regime of drastic purging, hot douches and a fruit and water diet. This she was assured would cure her swollen, aching joints. To effect the cure, she rose at 6 o'clock in the morning and, unadorned even by a fig leaf, entered an underground bath where her body was sprayed by a stream of scalding water, an experience which she claimed was 'a good rehearsal for purgatory'. After a week at Vichy, she was lighter and no doubt cleaner – but she still found difficulty in clenching her hands.

Many other notable figures have found relief in hot baths. Napoleon soothed his frayed nerves in a hot tub and, when the war with England broke out, spent 6 hours in his bath dictating letters to a relay of four secretaries. Lord Bacon extended the phlogistic cure still further. He took a 2-hour soak in a hot bath and followed it up by lying for 24 hours in a spiced cloth, then took an overall massage with scented body oils.

Today, the vogue for hot bathing remains, with the home sauna and bathroom jacuzzi taking over from the double garage and outdoor swimming pool as the favoured status symbol of the upward striving young executive. There is no doubt that wallowing in warm water is relaxing, as our forebears found, and can help to ease the discomfort of rheumatic pain, particularly when it is associated with muscular contraction. It functions by dilating the blood vessels and so enhancing the circulation to the affected area. This aids the healing of inflammation and speeds the removal of the waste products of muscle metabolism, which give rise to pain when they are allowed to accumulate in the bodies of tense muscles. Heat also helps to relax the muscle spasm and to raise the pain threshold.

It is possible to buy antirheumatic bath salts, but there is no evidence that these substances do anything to enhance the effectiveness of the bath itself, apart from colouring the water and supplying a therapeutic smell which may increase the cure's psychological potency. To obtain the benefit of a warm bath, all that is necessary is to linger and luxuriate in warm water for 15 to 20 minutes. During this time, try to relax as much as possible, listening perhaps to soothing music and resting your head on a folded towel or bath cushion. (Bath cushions were first introduced by King Louis XIII of France, who had them specially made when he switched from a traditional wooden tub to a sumptuous marble bath which proved too hard for the royal rump!)

Heat can also be applied by electric pads, hot water bottles, infra-red lamps and hot packs. Among farming communities in the UK, it was traditional to treat bouts of lumbago by ironing the back with a flat iron rubbed over a sheet of brown paper. This is a perfectly adequate technique, providing the paper is sufficiently thick and the iron is kept on the move. Heat is heat however it is applied and a painful back will derive as much benefit from sitting in front of an electric fire as from lying under an expensive heat lamp.

The advantage of an electric pad is that it can be applied directly to the painful area of the back. If it is lain on, however, it loses some of its effectiveness, since the blood vessels become compressed and the circulation reduced. Hot packs can be easily made by soaking a folded towel in hot water, squeezing it gently to remove the surplus water, and then applying it to the back. Their disadvantage is that they are messy and need to be resoaked every few minutes, but they can be very soothing, especially when administered by an attentive nurse or tender, caring spouse. Infra-red lamps provide a constant source of heat but are often difficult to beam on the required area of the back and can easily toast the skin if placed too close to the body. (When using them, remember that wave transmission observes the inverse square law, which means that halving the distance of a lamp from your body does not double but *quadruples* the heat striking the skin.)

Hot-water bottles are another convenient way of applying heat to the back. They hold about 2 pints (1 l) of water and can supply approximately 13,000 Calories of heat, half of which radiates to the body, the rest being dissipated in the air. They too should be used with care. Irreversible skin damage occurs if water at a temperature of 150° F (65° C) is placed in contact with the skin for even a few seconds. This nullifies the value of the treatment and can impair the circulation on a long-term basis. Patients often find it remarkable that I can sometimes pinpoint the exact location of their pain without detailed questioning or close examination. This is not difficult when the area is marked by a tell-tale mottling of the skin, caused by sitting too close to a heat lamp or by applying a bottle filled with excessively hot water. (A little surprise can also be caused by divining the positions that husbands and wives take in the evening on either side of the hearth. This too is done by spotting the mottling on the inside or outside of the wife's shins!)

People with a tendency to backache should take care to protect the circulation to their back. It is a widely held belief that lumbago comes from wearing damp clothes or sitting in a draught. This idea dates back to the days when disease was thought to be caused by the influence of the demon Lilith, the goddess of wind, who polluted the night air and invaded the bodies of sleeping children to give them abdominal cramps and 'wind'. This is why mothers sang protective spells to their children at night, which came to be known as Lullabies since they were intended to keep the demon lily-at-bay. But damp, draughts and chills are not nearly the bogies we take them to be and there is no evidence that they are a cause of rheumatic disease, even though they can at times be aggravating factors. The majority of men went through the World War 1, fighting in damp clothes and sleeping in water-logged trenches, without getting a trace of rheumatism. Likewise, when a team of doctors from the Medical Research Council compared the incidence of rheumatoid arthritis in the UK and Jamaica, they found that the disease actually occurred with equal frequency in the two countries, although the Jamaicans complained less, possibly because of their milder climate.

There is only one time when it *is* important to protect the spine from chilling and that is not while moving about and working actively but when the back muscles are subjected to static strain. You are unlikely to be stricken with lumbago when you are swimming in cold water or jogging around the park in a singlet and shorts in the depth of winter. This is because the rhythmical exercise keeps the circulation flowing through the back muscles in all but the most extreme conditions. (It is always advisable to 'warm up' for activities such as these to prevent the muscular strains which can occur before the muscle fibres are relaxed and the blood flow stimulated.) Problems arise when the muscles are used in conditions which subject them to a combination of postural tension and local chilling. A person drives a car on the motorway with the shoulders hunched over the steering wheel. Maintaining this crouched position keeps the muscles of the neck and shoulders in a state of unrelieved tension. This leads to a steady build-up of the acid waste products of muscle metabolism, which are not easily flushed away since the blood vessels are constricted by the tension in the surrounding muscle fibres. If it is a hot day, the motorist opens his offside window to get a breath of fresh air. This chills the skin and produces a reflex contraction of both the muscles and the deep, intramuscular blood vessels.

This adds to the build-up of metabolites and these act as chemical irritants of the fine nerve endings and can provoke a painful spasm of the muscles. This is a story I have heard on a number of occasions; it happens especially on hot, sunny days when the skin-cooling effect is exaggerated by the evaporation of sweat.

Similar events can give rise to bouts of acute lumbago. Here the precipitating activities are generally bending over weeding the garden or repairing a motor-car engine at a time when the back is damp with perspiration and exposed to a cold wind. These acute muscular spasms should be treated with heat and gentle exercise and prevented by wearing appropriate protective clothing. I agree with those experts who advise outdoor workers to keep their backs warm, especially when they are performing static work. Some, like Bath rheumatologist Dr George Kersley, advocate the wearing of thermal underwear and protective woollen body belts. 'In some people sensitivity to local chilling is of great significance', he explains, 'and clothing that doesn't strike cold – a warm belt ... or a sharp rub with a rough towel followed by exercises, if chilled, may avert an attack'.

But I am not in favour of excess mollycoddling. It is unwise to over-protect the body from the cold by living in permanently overheated offices and homes and wearing a constant cocoon of warm clothes, for this destroys the body's natural ability to protect itself from temperature change. Therefore I am equally well in agreement with another rheumatologist who said: 'Exposure of the skin avoiding local chilling not only acts as a powerful stimulant to metabolism, but assists in preventing that failure of reactivity of the superficial capillaries to change of temperature which, fostered by overclothing, is so often prodromal of rheumatic disease'. The ideal is to learn to live and work in varying climates, to avoid local chilling of the back while carrying out static work and to make judicious use of warmth as a therapeutic agent whenever the muscles are aching, tense or tired.

VERDICT *Heat is rarely a curative agent but can give considerable relief when back pain originates from muscular tension or stiffness. Various means are available for applying the heat – hot baths, infra-red lamps, warm packs, hot-water bottles and electric pads – some of which are more convenient to use than others. These techniques are equally effective and equally damaging when used injudiciously.*

20 Aye, There's The Rub

Massage is probably the oldest of all the healing arts. Even in his days in the primaeval forest, primitive man must have noticed that it was soothing to rub, pummel, press or stroke a painful, aching back. Later the work was carried out by specialists, who developed their manual dexterity by regular practice. In Japan, itinerant masseurs travelled from village to village, announcing their arrival in the market place by playing a few shrill notes on a flute. Today, such blatant professional advertising may be looked on with disfavour but the Japanese still value the services of their skilled masseurs, who may be found practising in well-equipped city clinics, as well as in outlying tea-houses and communal baths. In South America, the exotically garbed *paye*, the medicine-men of the ancient Indian tribes, administered massage to ward off rheumatism, making incantations as they did so to draw the pain into their own bodies. Now the businessmen of Rio de Janeiro have their back pains eased by white-coated physiotherapists, who may accompany their massage with a few muttered words about the weather, the cost of living, or the latest TV soap opera, but who no longer believe that spells can cast out the demons of disease.

Captain Cook, in the logbook of his third voyage, tells how he was stricken with lumbago and sciatica on the island of Tahiti. Unable to get relief, he sought the help of the islanders. They offered him the services of twenty native women, who were well versed in the craft of massage and manipulation. They, according to one report, 'squeezed him with both hands from head to foot, particularly where the pain was, until his bones cracked and his flesh was like a mummy'. The treatment lasted about 15 minutes and gave him considerable relief. A second dose that evening enabled him to sleep peacefully and the next day he was cured.

Every nation has its own tradition of massage, which mercifully is rarely as punishing as that given by the Tahitian maidens. In fact, massage is generally at its most effective when it is made soothing and relaxing. This lesson was learnt by Lucas-Championnière, a fashionable Parisian doctor who played a major part in putting manual treatment on a scientific footing in the nineteenth century by writing *The Treatment of*

Fractures by Massage and Mobilisation. Lucas-Championnière had watched the enormous success of an unqualified masseur who had built up a very lucrative practice in a neighbouring district of Paris. This man, with no medical training and using only the instruments of his hands, was earning more than most of the city's leading physicians. How did he do it? Several doctors asked him to divulge the formula of his success but always he refused. This was to remain his closely guarded secret. Then his son fell ill with peritonitis. Lucas-Championnière, the only sympathetic doctor he could find, operated on the lad at once and saved his life. The father was so grateful that he agreed to take the doctor into his confidence and tell him the principle which had enabled him to build up such a flourishing practice. 'I never hurt a patient', he said. That was the secret of his success!

When used in the treatment of back pain, massage serves two main functions. In the first place, it helps to relax muscle spasm. When the spine suffers a mechanical injury – a sprained joint, a trapped nerve or a damaged disc – the body's immediate response is to tense up. It wraps the back in a corset of protective muscle spasm. This is a worthy attempt to limit movement and prevent further damage but sometimes the cure is worse than the original disease. All the most painful conditions to which the human body is heir, such as angina, childbirth and renal colic, are associated with powerful muscle spasm. The same is true of the pain of acute lumbago, although here there is one major difference: the muscle cramps are often prolonged rather than spasmodic. The pains of angina, labour and renal colic disappear once you stop hurrying up a hill, are delivered of a baby, or pass the offending kidney stone, but the pain of lumbago can last as long as the underlying mechanical derangement persists. This can set up a self-perpetuating vicious circle for pain provokes protective muscle spasm, which in turn creates more pain and therefore initiates further muscle spasm. Relaxing massage is one way of interrupting this pernicious chain reaction. To achieve this end, the massage must be firm and steady. Anyone who has suffered repeated bouts of cramp in the calf will have discovered no doubt that there are two practical ways or relieving muscle spasm. One is to stretch the muscle's fibres by standing on the foot and drawing the toes towards the chin. The other is to grip the calf and apply firm manual pressure, which also inhibits the reflex muscle spasm. Both these principles – the stretching of the spastic muscle fibres and the firm, inhibitory pressure – should be applied to the muscles of the back when they are in a state of painful spasm. This can give considerable relief but naturally cannot be expected to correct any underlying structural disorder, which may need specialist treatment if it does not undergo spontaneous resolution.

In addition to its use as a palliative in cases of acute lumbago, massage is also highly effective in those cases of chronic backache which are associated with tender muscular lumps, sometimes referred to as trigger spots or fibrositic nodules. Over the years, these painful muscular knots have been something of a medical conundrum. At one time, they were thought to be due to toxic deposits or the haphazard laying-down of rheumatic crystals. Then someone took the trouble to subject the lumps to biochemical analysis. This failed to reveal the presence of any noxious substances or tissue inflammation. Some doctors were content to give the nodules a pseudo-scientific name. Since they could no longer use the term fibrositis, which means an inflammation of the fibrous tissues, they chose vague words like myalgia, which is Greek for muscle pain, or muscular rheumatism, which presumably means a settling of the evil humour 'rheum' in the muscles!

Other physicians, who placed more reliance on the negative biopsy findings than on the testimony of their patients or the evidence of their own fingers, began to doubt the existence of these muscular lumps. Any pain in a muscle, they decided, was either referred from elsewhere or was a figment of the imagination. This was a popular medical theory during my student days and I remember well the confusion caused in 1953 when Len Hutton, England's cricket captain, was stricken with fibrositis of the back in the middle of an important test match series. A doctor speaking on the radio voiced the thoughts of many sports fans when he said: 'With the fate of England hanging in the balance the problem of fibrositis has surely now become a matter of national importance. And to complicate matters, at the very time that England's captain is reputed to be suffering with this distressing, but fortunately never dangerous, malady, experts at the British Medical Association are heard to declare that no such thing exists. How can our fate and reputation as a cricketing nation depend upon the outcome of an illness that doesn't exist?'

In fact the existence of 'fibrositis' can be easily proved. The tender nodules can be felt by the doctor, studied by the physiologist and often spirited away by injections or skilled massage. There is no doubting their existence and no arguing away the pain they cause. The lumps are not rheumatic growths or toxic deposits but little bands of muscular tension and contraction. These can be brought on by a host of factors, such as injury, local chilling, postural strain, emotional tension, tiredness and muscular overuse. Some sites of the body are far more prone to develop these painful nodules than others. Figure 23 shows the danger areas for muscular trigger spots. It is based on a study carried out on patients referred to a clinic at the Oldchurch Hospital, Essex, because they had failed to respond to orthodox treatment for chronic backache. The patients' backs were probed with a rubber-tipped pen to bring to light their painful trigger spots. These were then treated by local injection. This produced rapid and complete relief of their chronic pain within

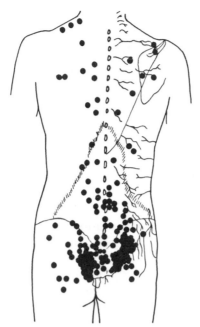

Figure 23 Trigger spots. The most common form of painful trigger spots.

2 weeks in 80 per cent of cases.

Massage can also help to remove these painful trigger spots. The technique is easily acquired by anyone who has the patience to learn and a genuine desire to help relieve the suffering of their loved ones, neighbours, workmates and friends.

PARTNER MASSAGE

Step One Get your patient to strip to the waist and lie face downwards either on a firm bed or on a suitably padded floor surface. Then spread a little oil over the surface of his or her back. This will enable you to move smoothly over the skin, applying firm pressure without dragging the tissues or causing unnecessary friction. Any handy lubricant – vegetable, animal or mineral – can be used for this purpose, such as baby oil, olive oil or sunflower seed oil. Or you may prefer to use one of the special body oils sold by herbalists and health food stores.

Step Two Kneel at your patient's head with your hands covering the shoulder blades and finger tips pointing towards the spine. Now run your hands slowly down the back, keeping your finger tips in the grooves on either side of the spine and applying firm pressure with your finger tips and the outside borders of both little fingers. As you reach the base of the spine, move your hands outwards across the crest of the pelvis until you reach the outside of the buttocks. Then, in one continuous

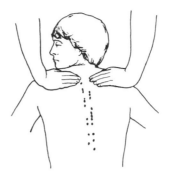

Figure 24 Partner massage. Step two.

movement, bring your hands backwards, gliding along your patient's flanks until you reach your starting position. Bend your trunk forward as you make the downward stroke and use your body weight to augment the pressure of your hands. Then gradually straighten up and ease the pressure as you make the recovery stroke. Repeat this complete cycle 10 times, as smoothly as possible. (See Figure 24.)

Step Three Kneel to your patient's side and place the tips of your fingers in the dimple just to the side of the base of the spine. Place one hand above the other for added pressure, then begin to make slow circular movements, moving outwards along the crest of the pelvis for about 2 in (5 cm) and then upwards in the furrows on the side of the spine. Travel upwards to the shoulder blades and then slowly backwards to the base of the spine, taking care to linger over spots where you detect tender muscular lumps and bumps. Then change position and repeat on the opposite side. (See Figure 25.)

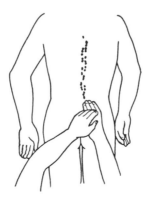

Figure 25 Partner massage. Step three.

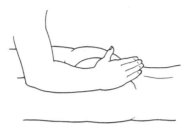

Figure 26 Partner massage. Step four.

Step Four The area where the gluteal muscles are attached to the rim of the pelvis is a common location for painful muscular nodules, yet the buttocks are often overlooked when giving back massage. To cover this region, kneel to one side of your patient and apply firm downward pressure with the heel of your hand just at the point where the muscles join the rim of the pelvis. Start about an inch from the midline and work the hands in a circular motion, moving slowly outwards along the line of the pelvic rim until you reach the upper aspects of the thighs. Do this 3 times, slowly and firmly and with particular attention to any tell-tale fibrositic nodules. Then repeat on the opposite side. (See Figure 26.)

Step Five End your session of back massage by repeating Step Two, only this time continue your downwards strokes to include the buttocks as well as the spinal muscles.

VERDICT Massage can give a measure of temporary relief in cases of acute lumbago and can help to overcome those cases of chronic back pain which arise mainly from fibrositic nodules. In the first case, the emphasis should be on firm, stretching movements to relax the protective muscle spasm. In the second case, the aim is to iron out the painful trigger spots with more localised, frictional massage. In both instances, the treatment is generally aided by the application of warmth in whatever form seems most convenient (see page 101).

21 A Source Of Irritation

There are few things more potent than smells to create a mood or evoke a memory. The smell of burning timber still reminds me of the camp fires I used to sit round years ago as a child; and the mouth-watering odour of doughnuts sizzling in the pan at our village baker's shop never fails to bring back memories of one particular seaside holiday when as a lad of nine or ten I used to present myself sharp on the dot of 11 o'clock at the local bakery to sample the first of their batch of freshly baked dough-nuts. A wave of nostalgia also comes over me whenever I get a whiff of wintergreen, for this takes my mind back to the crowded, convivial sport's changing rooms I used to frequent in my athletic youth.

This particular olfactory link is of great antiquity, for sportsmen and soldiers throughout the ages have employed a variety of aromatic oils to ease the aches in their weary limbs and fibrositic spines. This time-honoured practice is not without its medicinal value for the oils in tradi-tional use are all mild skin irritants. When applied to the surface of the body, they act as counter-irritants, reddening the skin, improving the circulation to the treated area and setting up a barrage of mild, nerve sensations which helps to block the perception of pain from deeper structures. When Roman soldiers suffered from lumbago, they were beaten with a switch of stinging nettles, an uncomfortable cure which combined the therapeutic effectiveness of a hot bath with that of an intensive course of paraspinal acupuncture! A few centuries later, back-pain sufferers were given the red-ant cure, a container filled with the insects being placed in contact with the affected part of their bodies just long enough for it to become inflamed with their chemical-laden stings.

Charles Dickens was a frequent sufferer from muscular rheumatism, possibly because of the postural strain of his occupation or from the stress produced by his compulsive addiction to work. He derived great benefit from using a counter-irritant cream made from oil of wintergreen. Today the chemists' shelves are filled with endless proprietary liniments, lotions and salves, all offering to ease rheumatic pain. Most are based on ancient herbal remedies, but a few offer more up-to-date 'scientific' ingredients. One, for instance, contains adrenalin to dilate the blood

110

vessels. Tests of this cream some years ago showed it to be less effective than the old remedies it was intended to replace. When rubbed into the skin, it had a soothing effect, but this was no greater than when the body was anointed with ordinary cold cream. Obviously it was the massage which gave the relief and not the medicament itself.

To have a therapeutic effect, an embrocation must give rise to some degree of superficial discomfort and skin irritation. For maximum benefit it should be employed after a preliminary warming of the skin. This was appreciated by Galen, the great Greek physician, who, when working in Rome, recommended that gladiators in preparation for exercise should be rubbed until they were red and then anointed with oils. Red flannel, worn in close contact with the back, was another popular remedy for lumbago. This had some scientific validity in the days of our great grandparents, for red flannel was originally obtained by dyeing the raw woollen cloth in an extract of madder root, a substance which was a powerful counter-irritant as well as an effective colourant. Today, when synthetic dyes are used, there is no point in wrapping the skin in red flannel, unless of course it has been specially impregnated with a counter-irritant substance.

Another cure favoured by our forebears was an alcohol friction rub. When they suffered a bout of lumbago, they generally drank copious quantities of warm water to flush their kidneys and had an alcohol rub to enhance the circulation to their backs. Now the order is reversed. When we have a spell of back pain, we tend to wallow in the warm water and swallow the alcohol. This is almost certainly a more effective use of these valuable resources, for a hot bath *will* help to relax and improve the circulation to tense muscle groups, whereas flushing the kidneys with draughts of warm water does nothing to ease rheumatic pain. And whereas alcohol is a useful sedative and muscle relaxant when taken internally, it does nothing helpful when rubbed on the surface of the body, except to act as a skin cleanser.

Over the years, a number of substances have been used for their counter-irritant effect, such as methyl salicylate, which was originally obtained from oil of wintergreen but is now often made by chemical synthesis. Menthol, one of the active ingredients of peppermint oil, is both a counter-irritant and mild surface anaesthetic. The same applies to camphor and clove oil, which are often used to ease toothache pains. Capsicum, turpentine oil, eucalyptus and mustard oil are other powerful and frequently used counter-irritants. Most popular liniments and salves contain a mixture of these ingredients. Sloan's Liniment®, the athlete's stand-by, contains turpentine, camphor, methyl salicylate and capsicum. The formula of a deep-heating rub called Mentholatum® includes menthol, methyl salicylate, eucalyptus oil and turpentine oil. And one called Ben-Gay Lotion®, which started out in life as Dr Bengue's Balsam, 'A wonderful remedy for rheumatism, gout, neuralgia', is made from menthol and salicylate.

There is little to choose between these remedies, which should be selected on grounds of cost and aroma – either most pleasing or least obnoxious according to the acuity of your sense of smell! Only two safeguards should be observed: since the creams are generally poisonous and highly irritating, they should not be taken internally and should not be applied to sensitive or damaged skin.

VERDICT *A useful, and generally safe, way of easing mild muscular aches and pains – providing you can stand the smell! Unlikely to be of any value in treating sciatic or severe back pains.*

22 A Painful Matter

As soon as man discovered the medicinal value of herbs, he began a quest which continues today – the search for the perfect analgesic drug, the remedy which will kill pain but produce no untoward side effects. The North American Indians deadened their pain by taking extracts of the bark of the willow tree (*Salix*). This contained natural analgesic substances which, because of their origin, came to be called salicylates. Nowadays, Americans ease their back pains and headaches by taking a derivative of this substance known as acetylsalicylic acid or aspirin. This they swallow at the rate of 16 billion tablets a year. In the hot countries bordering on the Mediterranean Sea, a popular narcotic was derived from the seeds of a species of poppy known as *Papaver somniferum*. These contained large quantities of opium and were either chewed or smoked in special pipes. From this source, we derive powerful pain-killers such as codein and morphine.

Today the pharmacists' shops are filled with a bewildering range of drugs which all offer to ease the pain of backache and sciatica. Which brand should one choose? All have pain-relieving properties and all are capable of causing undesirable side effects. But then exactly the same could be said of tablets made from sugar and starch, which contain no active ingredients whatsoever. These dummy pills, or placebos, have been shown to relieve back pain in about 35 per cent of cases. One doctor has also written a paper in the *Journal of the American Medical Association*, describing the side effects of taking these phony drugs, which embraces over thirty-five different toxic symptoms. Another has reported cases of patients who have even become addicted to their placebos!

The response we show to drugs depends on our faith and expectations, as well as on the pharmacological properties of the remedy itself. Trials show that placebos are most effective if they are coloured red, yellow or brown. Their potency is also greater if they have a bitter taste and if they are unusually large or small. The confidence of the person prescribing a dummy remedy is another crucial factor. One test revealed that, when the placebos were handed out by a non-committal nurse, they had a success rate of only 25 per cent whereas, when exactly the same placebo was offered by an enthusiastic doctor, the success rate soared to 70 per cent!

When we are anxious and in pain, the confident bearing of a healer can be as curative as the treatment he prescribes. As I know from experience, back pain of long duration can disappear the moment a patient arrives for treatment. How sheepish patients sometimes feel when they are forced to admit that the agonising pain which they have had for months has miraculously disappeared the very morning of their initial consultation! With old patients, the mere fact of making an appointment for treatment is occasionally enough to effect a cure, such is the power of faith and trust.

Personality factors also influence the way we react to analgesic drugs. Some people have lower pain thresholds than others, especially when they are anxious, tired or depressed. Others tend to react more keenly to all forms of sensory stimulation. This was demonstrated in a series of elegant experiments conducted by Harvard University psychologist Asenath Petrie. She took a series of blindfolded subjects and asked them to use their right hand to estimate the width of various blocks of wood and their left hand to mark off the same thickness on a tapered measuring bar. Some peoples' perception was pretty accurate but a number consistently exaggerated the width of the blocks, while a further group tended to underestimate their size. Additional tests showed that the 'augmenters' were generally introverts who perceived everything, including pain, more keenly than their fellows. The 'reducers' on the other hand were normally active extroverts with a high pain threshold. These two groups also showed a variation in their response to medication, the 'augmenters' being highly responsive to drugs such as aspirin and alcohol at a dosage which had little influence on the more stolid 'reducers'.

Recent research has shown that we have far more control over our pain response than was previously thought. People who learn to relax are far better able to cope with pain than those who hold themselves tense. So too are those who can distract their attention to other things rather than constantly focusing their mind on their aches and pains. Experience of suffering also helps to make pain easier to bear. This explains why people who have never had a day's illness often make the most difficult patients. They find it hard to accept that *they* should be smitten with something as disabling as backache or sciatica. Even a passing twinge can seem like a monstrous calamity to these virgin sufferers.

Trials carried out by psychologists at Pennsylvania State University have revealed that our ability to withstand pain grows with repeated exposure. We can inoculate ourselves against pain, just as we can vaccinate ourselves against smallpox or diptheria. The Pennsylvanian trials made use of student volunteers, who were all given a simple pain tolerance test that involved holding their hands as long as possible in freezing water. The students were then divided into five groups. The

114

first received no treatment whatsoever and was used as a control group. The second was given general information about the psychological mechanisms of pain and advice on how to ease the anxiety which normally accompanies it. The third group was taught specific pain-relieving techniques, such as relaxation therapy, and distraction methods which switched the subjects' attention from any pain they were experiencing to conjured-up scenes of tranquillity and ease. The fourth was told that practice would inure them to the pain and were encouraged to build up their resistance by repeatedly dipping their hands in icy water. The fifth had the benefit of both the practice exposures and the training in pain-relieving techniques. When the students resubmitted themselves to the ice-water test, it was found that the last group could keep their hands in the water much longer than any other group and reported far less discomfort when doing so. Lesser improvements were shown by the third and fourth groups, which proves that we can train ourselves to withstand pain.

The body has its own method of coping with pain, which is ours to use and which gives us support, particularly in times of crisis. Research has revealed that the body is capable of manufacturing natural opiates, known as endorphins, which have the same sedative effect on the brain's pain centres as morphine. There is some evidence that we can increase the output of these neuro-hormones by an act of will (see page 144). Certainly tests show that the effectiveness of taking placebos is related to the release of endorphins and it is probable that the same applies to the induction of states of analgesia by hypnotic suggestion. In the heat of the battle, when animals are savaged by predators or boxers injured in the ring, they may feel remarkably little pain, because their bodies are flooded with endorphins. At times, they may even feel euphoric, because they are on a chemical 'high'. Lord Raglan was so alive and alert after his arm had been amputated without an anaesthetic after the Battle of Waterloo that he cheerfully called out to the medical orderlies: 'Here, bring that arm back; there is a ring my wife gave me on the finger'.

We can undoubtedly increase our natural ability to withstand pain, but there are many times when it is comforting to have the assistance of artificial aids. Drugs can often provide this welcome support, easing pain, allaying inflammation, inducing sleep and relaxing painful muscle spasm. The drug treatment of back-pain syndromes is best carried out under the supervision of a doctor and is described, in outline only, on page 135. For home use, I normally recommend only two drugs. Both are powerful remedies, with side effects which are by now well documented and understood. The first is aspirin, used partly as an anti-inflammatory agent but more especially as a painkiller. The second is alcohol, which also has analgesic properties but which is most valuable in its role as a muscle relaxant. Aspirin should be taken only when the pain is severe. For adults, the maximum recommended dose is two 5-grain tablets every 4 hours. The drug normally begins to take effect after about 30 minutes, and generally loses its pain-numbing properties after 2 or 3 hours. As it is a powerful gastric irritant, aspirin should not be used by peptic ulcer sufferers and should always be taken either with, or immediately after, meals. Even with these precautions, it is estimated that two-thirds of people who take three to four aspirin tablets a day suffer gastro-intestinal bleeding. If this is severe, the stools may become darkened by the presence of iron from the broken-down blood pigment. This is a warning sign to stop taking aspirin and switch to a drug which is kinder to the gastric tract, such as codeine.

Alcohol is a useful, multi-purpose drug, as many back-pain sufferers have discovered. It eases pain, allays anxiety and also helps to relax muscle spasm. This explains why inebriates fall so easily when they trip over their shoe laces or bend down to retrieve the house key from its traditional hiding place under the front door mat. If they continue to drink beyond this point, their muscles are rendered so totally relaxed that they give the appearance of being 'paralytic'. A lesser degree of this state, induced by drinking a double or treble Scotch, can help to ease the painful muscle spasms of acute backache and sciatica. This is a handy remedy to take before retiring to bed, when it can help to induce a restful night's sleep, but it should never be taken when driving or handling dangerous machinery, since it can play havoc with co-ordination and reflex responses. This was proved by Larry Adler, the world-famous mouth-organ virtuoso. He was scheduled to play a concert in Manchester with the Hallé Orchestra. On the night of the performance, Adler was stricken with a bout of backache which was so severe that he asked his conductor, Sir John Barbirolli, if he would object to him sitting down to play. The conductor readily agreed but asked him if he would first try his personal backache cure. In Sir John's dressing room, Adler was given two stiff cognacs. 'After drinking these brandies you will feel no pain', Adler was assured. This promise came true. Unfortunately the soloist was not warned that the alcohol would also ruin his reflexes and cause him to give what he later confessed was his worst performance ever. His only salvation was that he was playing an entirely new work – the Vaughan Williams' *Romance for Mouthorgan, Piano and Strings* – so nobody in the packed concert hall knew that he was playing it wrong!

VERDICT *Pain is a subjective symptom, the experience of which can be modified by drugs and also by experience, relaxation, distraction, stress, auto-suggestion, faith and sheer determination. The two safest and most effective medicines for back-pain sufferers to administer themselves are aspirin and alcohol, but even these familiar remedies have powerful side effects and should be used with discrimination and care.*

23 Getting The Needle

Acupuncture has been a popular form of treatment in the Orient for over 4,000 years. According to one legend, the therapy arose by accident after soldiers reported that, when their flesh was punctured with arrows, they sometimes lost their awareness of chronic pain elsewhere in their bodies. Others believe that the system had its origins in a totally different chance experience. They tell how a worker, suffering from severe headache, dropped a heavy stone upon his foot. Immediately his toes began to throb with pain, but as they did so his headache disappeared as if by a miracle. There is a certain ring of truth about this tale for, even today, acupuncurists stimulate a spot close to the big toe to relieve headaches and migraine and, for years, the early acupuncurists stimulated their patient's skin not with a metal needle as they do today, but with a pointed lump of stone known as a *bian shi* or stone-piercer.

Whatever the exact origin of the art of acupuncture, it quickly became a major resource of Eastern healers, and so it remains today, with China claiming a million registered acupuncturists and Japan a further 50,000.

In recent years, the West has taken a greatly increased interest in this ancient form of healing. Doctors throughout the world have published reports of operations successfully carried out under acupuncture analgesia. Russian scientists tell of cases of bed-wetting and sexual impotence and frigidity cured by electro-acupuncture. Even more remarkable are the testimonies of the medical teams who have visited China and witnessed cases of childhood deafness completely cured by acupuncture. Less dramatic perhaps, and therefore less well publicised, is the evidence that acupuncture can relieve backache and sciatica. In 1972, the Consumers' Association quizzed a group of over 200 of their members who had visited an acupuncturist. Most had been suffering from lumbago, sciatica or non-specified rheumatism, for which doctors had given them pain-killing drugs. They found the insertion of the needles caused little or no discomfort and were generally pleased with the result of the treatment, which 70 per cent said had relieved their pain. Nine years later, a team of doctors at St Bartholomew's Hospital, London, under the leadership of Professor Michael Bender, carried out a more controlled trial of the use of acupuncture in the treatment of chronic back pain. They reported a similar cure rate of 70–75 per cent.

In the past, doctors found it difficult to believe in the efficacy of acupuncture, because it did not fit in with their traditional concepts about the anatomy and working of the human body. They could not accept that diseases could be diagnosed by palpating twelve distinct pulses at the wrist or that the sum total of human illness was due to an imbalance between the opposing life forces of the *yin* and *yang*. Likewise, they found it impossible to place any special significance on the 1,000 named acupuncture points and could not believe in the circulation of the *ch'i* along the twelve meridians, the pathways which acupuncturists believe run up and down the body on either side. Nevertheless, they were forced to concede that acupuncture could, and very often did, relieve pain. How could this be explained?

Recent research work has brought to light two possible explanations for the efficacy of acupuncture. As a contributor to the *Journal of the American Medical Association* concluded, after reviewing the available evidence and pouring scorn on some of the system's more fanciful notions: 'The evidence now available is sufficient to place this age-old Chinese healing art, modernized to US standards, on a solid scientific base'. Experiments revealed that the brain is capable of producing its own pain-killing drugs, the endorphins, which have a very similar effect to morphine. The output of these natural opiates has been shown to increase when the skin is stimulated with either acupuncture needles, electric impulses or deep finger pressure. This helps to raise the pain threshold, sometimes to a quite dramatic extent. Tests at Peking Medical College have demonstrated that rabbits are able to stand twice as much pain if they are given a supportive dose of finger acupuncture or acupressure. (Their skins are too sensitive to stand needling.)

Investigations into the mechanism of pain perception have introduced another possible explanation for the effectiveness of acupuncture analgesia. Most doctors today subscribe to the 'gate control theory' of pain, formulated by Professor Ronald Melzack of McGill University, Montreal, and Professor Patrick Wall of University College, London. This holds that certain nerve cells in the spinal cord have a modifying influence on the pain impulses travelling to the brain, being able either to intensify them or diminish them. According to this theory, the effect of the needling of the skin is to set up a steady barrage of nerve impulses which effectively blocks the passage of painful stimuli to the brain, in the same way that a radio broadcast can be 'jammed'. Possibly both these mechanisms of pain relief are operating when acupuncture needles are inserted and twiddled in the flesh, when deep finger pressure is applied or when tiny piles of powdered herbs are burnt on the skin (moxibustion). In either case, the technique would appear to be general in its effect rather than specific. In this case, there is no need to apply treatment to specific acupuncture points or along any particular meridian. Any spot on the surface of the body should be as effective as another. This has been proved in practice, for trials in China and Sweden have shown that the increase in pain threshold is not localised to one particular area but is uniform throughout the entire body. This makes a nonsense of the stand of the acupuncturist who, when asked to justify his charge of £20 for ten minutes' needling of a patient's ear, submitted a second bill:

For poking ear with pin	.50p
For knowing where to poke	£19.50
	£20.00

All the available evidence suggests that any spot on the ear could have been used with equal benefit.

If pain relief is provided by drugs, it needs to be given several times a day. The same is likely to be true of acupuncture analgesia. This can be done quite simply at home by applying firm, intermittent pressure to any convenient site on the body. One suitable spot is the fleshy web between the thumb and index finger, a favourite acupuncture point known as *Ho Ku*. Other handy sites for acupressure are the ear lobe and the *quenlum*, a traditional pressure point at the back of the heel just above the Achilles tendon. Rapid pinching of these spots, at a frequency about two nips per second, has been shown to raise the pain threshold considerably and to produce a significant increase in the output of pain-relieving endorphins.

Alternatively you could try biting your lower lip, a method of jamming pain perception which probably has as long a history in the West as acupuncture in the East.

VERDICT *Although in no sense a cure, acupuncture can be a valuable aid in easing the severity of back pains and sciaticas. From the currently available evidence it would appear that simple techniques of acupressure, suitable for self use, are just as effective in raising the pain threshold as the more complicated and costly techniques of needling used by professional acupuncturists.*

24 Cold Cures

A study of medical history should be an essential part of every doctor's training, if not to extend their therapeutic armamentarium then at least to imbue them with a reasonable sense of humility. Even a cursory look through the writings of the early physicians is enough to confirm Solomon's contention that 'there is no new thing under the sun'. This is particularly true of the use of ice packs and cold sprays in the treatment of acute back pains and sciaticas, a remedy of considerable antiquity which is still in use today.

The Greeks generally set their healing temples by the outlet of mountain springs, so that the sick could bathe in their cold, soothing water. In Rome, the life of the Emperor Augustus was saved by the application of cold compresses, which were one of the few truly effective treatments of the day. In mediaeval England, Christian pilgrims in search of healing bathed in the ice-cold wells at Walsingham and Holywell. At St Ann's Well, Buxton, the elderly discarded their crutches after dipping their rheumatic limbs in the spa's freezing waters.

By the start of the eighteenth century, the cold-bath remedy had left the realms of folk magic and become a recognized medical treatment, particularly for acute rheumatic pains. Staffordshire farm labourers who strained their spines while toiling in the fields were encouraged to bathe their backs in cold water drawn from the well at Willowbridge. In Lichfield, the eminent physician Sir John Floyer went one stage further. He built two baths side by side for the use of his rheumatic patients, an upper one for ladies which drained into a lower one reserved for men. These were fed by a spring a mile outside the town, so chosen because it provided the iciest water Sir John could find after scouring the vicinity and making exhaustive tests with a thermometer. John Wesley was another great advocate of cold baths, which he recommended as a cure for virtually every malady from hydrophobia to the falling sickness. On one of his horseback journeys he met a lady – a Mrs Bates of Leicester – who was suffering from crippling sciatica. After following the preacher's advice for 4 weeks, and taking liberal quantities of cold water both inside and out, her agonising pains disappeared.

During the century which followed, the cold-water cure became thoroughly institutionalized, being dispensed with enormous fervour at innumerable spas throughout Europe. (A rough count in 1842 showed that Germany alone had over fifty hydrotherapy centres.) The high priest of the cult was undoubtedly Vincenz Priessnitz, the ambitious farmer's boy who built a spa at Gräfenberg, high in the Silesian mountains. Here the rich and famous were sponged, showered, hosed, douched, plunge-bathed, wet-packed and dosed with endless glasses of spring water. One British doctor visiting Gräfenberg claimed that, during his stay, he had taken 500 cold baths, 2,400 sitz baths, lain in wet sheets for 480 hours and drunk 3,500 tumblers of cold water. Far from being intimidated by this stoic treatment, the doctor was so impressed by its curative powers that he returned to England and immediately took a lease on the Crown Hotel, Malvern. This he turned into a watering establishment along the Priessnitz lines and renamed it Gräfenberg House. From these simple beginnings, Malvern blossomed into an elegant spa town, a centre of healing for sufferers from rheumatism, back pain and sciatica, and a place of pilgrimage for eminent Victorians, such as Tennyson, Dickens, Carlyle and the delicate but determined Florence Nightingale. Mean-while, in Bavaria, a parish priest, Father Sebastian Kneipp, was trying the water cure on his parishioners. Such was his success that his little town of Wörishofen soon became inundated with health-seekers from the entire European continent. One government official consulted Father Kneipp after he had suffered for 3 months with severe sciatic pain running down the back of his left leg from buttock to foot. All orthodox treatments had failed to relieve the pain, which had not been touched by the repeated baths that he had taken as hot as he could bear. In despera-tion, the bureaucrat decided to make the uncomfortable trek to Wörishofen. Here he was told to discard all thoughts of steaming soaks and switch instead to douching his back with twice-daily effusions of cold water. On this spartan regime, he showed immediate progress. After the first day's treatment he slept for 4 hours, the best night's rest he had experienced since the trouble started. At the end of 4 weeks, his pain had been reduced to an irritating twinge. After 6 weeks, he was fully cured.

Cases like these might be dismissed as mere mumbo jumbo, ever-recurring examples of the amazing power of human credulity and faith to override the faculty of reason. Yet it is unwise to dismiss folk cures which have stood the test of time without fair appraisal for, if they have survived several centuries of clinical trial, it is highly likely that they are grounded on sound physiological principles. Can this be true of the cold water cure? Can cold applications genuinely ease the pain of lumbago and sciatica and, if so, how do they work?

Mothers throughout time have used a cold hand to soothe their

121

children's fevered brows. Footballer trainers have coped with their players' painful knocks and bruises armed only with a 'magic' cold sponge. These are simple examples of cryo-analgesia. The medical profession began to sit up and take a serious scientific interest in this subject only in 1902, when it was reported that cold, provoked by the evaporation of an ethyl chloride spray, could relieve the pain of severe earache. Other doctors found they could use this technique with equal success to ease the pain of menstruation, renal colic or acute heart attacks. The ethyl chloride spray proved particularly effective in the treatment of acute lumbago. In fact, Dr Maurice Ellis, consultant surgeon in charge of the casualty department of Leeds General Infirmary, considered that this was its most effective use. He had patients brought into his emergency wards locked with pain and bent sideways with muscle spasm. After treating their backs with the cooling spray for 20 to 30 seconds, he noted a dramatic lessening in their deformity and pain. As he reported in 1961 in a major article in the *British Medical Journal*: 'During the next few minutes the return of the normal lumbar curve can be seen to take place under the eyes of the surgeon, together with the disappearance of the scoliosis. When the patient turns to lie on his back he will admit that the acute pain has gone'. Many of his colleagues performed similar feats. But the remedy, which seemed to offer a miracle cure for acute back pain, was not without its problems. Ethyl chloride is a volatile liquid, toxic, flammable and even explosive when mixed with air in certain proportions. It is also an anaesthetic and, since the gas it forms is heavier than air, it tends to be inhaled by patients lying in the prone position, with unfortunate effects. To overcome these snags, Dr Janet Travell, physical medicine consultant to the White House during President Kennedy's days in office, experimented with a number of other liquids of low boiling point which were equally capable of cooling the skin when they evaporated. After much trial and error, a Philadelphian firm of pharmaceutical chemists – Smith, Kline and French Laboratories – elected to use a mixture of fluoromethanes. These they packed in metal pressurized cannisters, similar to those used in aerosol hair lacquers or household fly sprays. These cooling sprays are available at pharmacies under a variety of trade names.

An alternative way of chilling the skin is by using a cold pack. Nowadays, these usually consist of sealed plastic bags filled with hydrated silicate gels. These packs have two major advantages: they are easily moulded to fit the shape of the back and can be slipped back into the freezing compartment of the fridge whenever they thaw out and then be reused. A large pack of frozen peas can be used in exactly the same way. These make excellent and very economical cold packs, since the contents can be eaten once the treatment is over, providing they have not been removed from the fridge for more than a few moments at a time.

When cold packs and sprays were first employed to ease the pain of severe muscle spasm, it was assumed that they acted as local anaesthetics, deadening the skin and so blocking the passage of painful stimuli. This theory was quickly discarded when it was found that the treatment did not have to anaesthetize the skin to be effective. In fact, tests showed that, if the cooling was taken to excess, so that the skin was genuinely numbed, the pain was likely to be exacerbated rather than relieved. Refrigerant treatment works because it provides a form of counter-irritation. Far from damping down the flow of nerve impulses, it actually initiates a barrage of stimuli which is so strong that it blocks the perception of pain in the brain. This in turn interrupts the pain-tension-pain cycle and can bring about rapid relief of the protective muscle spasm which is generally so prominent a feature of attacks. When the treatment is successful, it can melt the tension accompanying acute back pain like snow in the noonday sun, straightening backs which have previously been twisted like corkscrews. There are three practical points to be observed in the application of refrigerant therapy, the relevance of which can now be appreciated:

☆ The back must be chilled sufficiently to trigger off the maximum possible release of nerve stimuli without giving rise to actual pain.

☆ The chilling must not be so intense or so prolonged that it deadens the skin, for this will render the treatment ineffective and may also cause frostbite damage to the superficial tissues.

☆ Intermittent applications of cold – lasting ½–1 minute – are generally more effective than continuous exposure, since their abruptness and regular interruption increases the intensity of the stimulation.

To apply the cold cure, expose the victim's back and lay him or her face downwards with the abdomen supported by one or two pillows, so that the hollow in the back is obliterated. This position helps to lessen the pressure on the emerging spinal nerves and also serves to stretch the back's powerful erector spine muscles. Then apply a purpose-built cold pack or pack of frozen peas to the affected portion of the spine. Keep this in contact with the skin for 30 seconds, then remove it for 10 seconds. Repeat this alternating process for 3 to 5 minutes, then leave the patient to relax. If the treatment is successful, it can be repeated three or four times a day. When a cooling spray is used, adopt the same posture but follow the directions for use printed on the cannister.

VERDICT Cold applications are of little use in the treatment of chronic backache, but can sometimes give marked and rapid relief of the pain and muscle spasm accompanying acute back injuries. Providing the skin is not damaged by overchilling, the treatment has no adverse side effects. Where cost is an important consideration the cold should be applied by means of a cold pack, which is just as effective as the more expensive and rapidly exhausted cold sprays sold in the pharmacists' shops.

25 The Anti-Lumbago Diet

One way of assessing the scientific standing of a book about rheumatism or backache is to measure the space it allots to dietary cures. If it is a serious scientific textbook, it will probably not contain a single word to suggest that nutritional factors could play any part whatsoever in the cause or relief of spinal disorders. If it is a book of folklore, it will be crammed from cover to cover with herbal remedies for lumbago and anti-acid diets which never fail to relieve arthritis, sciatica and degenerative back problems.

Many of the dietary cures for lumbago are little more than witches' brews of crushed ants and boiled sheep's eyes. Typical of this genre was the remedy which appeared in a book published in 1753. This consisted of a posset made by curdling a quart of boiled milk with 3 pints of beer, strained through a layer of horse dung! The more revolting the concoction the more effective it was thought to be and the higher its alcohol content the greater the likelihood that, even if it didn't actually cure spinal problems, it would at least make the aches and pains a trifle easier to bear. One of the most effective ingredients of these ancient country cures, which was never listed in the recipes themselves, was faith. This remains true today. In recent decades one of the most popular dietary regimes for rheumatism has been cider vinegar, a folk cure which hails from the State of Vermont and which was popularised by Dr D.C. Jarvis in his best-selling book *Arthritis and Common Sense*. People want to believe that they can cure their rheumatic ailments by pouring remedies down their gullet. 'We are what we eat' we are often told but, with the great mass of spinal problems, it would be far more accurate to say 'We are what we do'. Dr Jarvis advised his patients to sip slowly after every meal a glass of water containing 2 teaspoonsful of cider vinegar and an equal measure of honey. The theory he advanced to support this cure was that the cider vinegar augmented the natural acidity of the stomach. This aided the process of digestion and helped to kill off bacteria lurking in the digestive tract. It is difficult to see what this could do to relieve any of the common rheumatic disorders and a trifle naive to expect that a few drops of mild acetic acid could make any appreciable difference to the process of digestion, especially as the stomach normally contains acid enough of its own.

Ironically, during the years when Dr Jarvis was trying to encourage Americans to increase the acidity of their intestinal contents, nature-cure practitioners in the UK were engaged in an equally vigorous campaign to encourage Britons to do exactly the reverse! All forms of rheumatism, they claimed, were due to hyperacidity of the blood. So they placed their patients on an alkaline diet. The commonest prescription was to exist on a fresh fruit diet for at least a week. During this time, three meals a day were taken, consisting exclusively of ripe apples, pears and any other fresh, juicy fruits which happened to be in season. The only drinks permitted were pure water or unsweetened natural fruit juice; tea, coffee and alcohol were banned. The urine of people existing on this diet invariably became less acid. This was taken as a sign that the acidity of the blood was being reduced, thereby reducing the patient's tendency to rheumatism. There were two faults in this argument. In the first place, with the notable exception of gout, there is no evidence of any link between hyperacidity and any of the rheumatic diseases. Secondly, changes in the diet makes no difference whatsoever to the acidity of the blood, except during extreme starvation. This is merciful for, when changes in the acidity of the blood *do* occur, in diseases such as diabetes and kidney failure, they have an invariably catastrophic effect on bodily metabolism.

This is not to doubt the value of nature-cure regimes or all-fruit diets, from which many rheumatic sufferers appear to have derived considerable benefit, but merely to suggest that, if they show improvement on this regime, it is not due to a change in the acidity of their blood. A far more likely explanation is that, on this diet, they enjoy a beneficial increase in Vitamin C intake. Some years ago the Mayo Clinic in the USA advised rheumatic sufferers to take regular doses of a cocktail of mixed, freshly pressed fruit juices. Many patients showed an encouraging response to this simple remedy (see page 140). This may have been due to their increased consumption of Vitamin C, which is known to play an important role in the metabolism of collagen, the basic raw material from which the body's connective tissues – skin, ligaments, joint cartilages and synovial membranes – are formed. Vitamin C is a vital constituent of the cement substance which binds together the cells forming the lining membranes of the blood vessels and the smooth synovium coating the insides of joint capsules. This is why bruising, bleeding gums and painful swelling of the joints are cardinal symptoms of gross Vitamin C deficiency states, known clinically as scurvy. It is possible that a dietary lack of Vitamin C, not severe enough to cause the full-blown syndrome of scurvy, could nevertheless be sufficient to increase the fragility of the synovial membrane lining the joints and to hamper the rate of joint tissue repair after injury.

Recent research work has pointed to another possible protective role of Vitamin C. An important component of all connective tissues is a substance known as hyaluronic acid. This strengthens the synovial membranes of the joints and checks the spread of infectious agents and inflammatory substances such as histamine. When hyaluronic acid is in short supply, there is an increased risk of arthritis or bleeding into the joint. Painful arthritic swelling of the joints can also result from an excessive activity of hyaluronidase, the naturally occurring substance which is responsible for the breakdown of hyaluronic acid in the body. This may occur as a direct result of Vitamin C lack, because research work carried out by Professor J.W.T. Dickerson of the Department of Biochemistry, Surrey University, has revealed that Vitamin C inhibits the action of hyaluronidase. Troubles may therefore arise from a complex sequence of events, in which an initial shortage of Vitamin C leads to an overactivity of hyaluronidase, which in turn causes an excessive breakdown of hyaluronic acid. This weakens the lining membranes of the joints and makes them excessively vulnerable to injuries, infections and inflammation.

Just how important this mechanism is in the production of joint pain is not yet clear but it is known that many people are subsisting on diets deficient in Vitamin C. In the UK, the recommended minimum allowance of Vitamin C is set at 30 mg per day, whereas medical authorities in the USA advise a daily ration of at least 60 mg. I am happier if my patients get twice or three times this level, say 100–200 mg per day. This particularly applies to those who smoke, who are under stress, recovering from an illness or taking drugs which depress the level of Vitamin C in the blood, such as aspirin, tetracycline antibiotics or hormone pills containing oestrogen. An intake of 30 mg of Vitamin C a day is probably sufficient to prevent scurvy but it is almost certainly not enough to maintain optimum health. And yet about one in six families in the UK are believed to be getting less than the minimum suggested ration of 30 mg a day, a figure which rises to an alarming one in two in February and March.

If there is such a thing as an anti-lumbago diet, it should be one which contains generous helpings of Vitamin C. This can be achieved by eating some fresh citrus fruit every day, together with plenty of salads and lightly cooked green vegetables. As a rough guide, a medium-sized orange contains 50 mg of Vitamin C, a glass of orange juice 93 mg, a cupful of coleslaw 50 mg and a medium-sized tomato 35 mg.

A diet designed for back-pain sufferers should also contain an adequate allowance of calcium and Vitamin D, the nutrients which are essential for the formation of strong, healthy bones. As we age, we suffer a gradual diminution of skeletal strength; our bones lose some of their mineral content and become progressively thinner in texture and more prone to

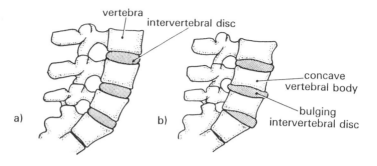

Figure 27 Vertebral column: a) normal b) degenerative.

fracture. This decline is particularly rapid in women after the menopause, because oestrogen, the main female hormone, plays a role in preventing bone loss. The term osteoporosis is used to describe an exaggerated loss of bone texture. This condition predisposes to fractures and contributes to the degenerative changes found in so many elderly spines. When they grow too weak to carry the imposed weight of the body, the vertebrae tend to collapse and become wedge-shaped, causing a stooping of the spine generally referred to as senile kyphosis. Sometimes the vertebrae are so weak that they cannot resist the bulging pressure of the intervertebral discs. In this case the vertebral bodies collapse inwards, as shown in Figure 27. One immediate result of the vertebral collapse and increased stoop is a loss of height of 1 or even 2 in (2.5 to 5 cm). Normally our height is virtually the same as our arm span but, when osteoporotic changes shrink the spine, we become somewhat simian in our dimensions, with an arm span noticeably greater than our height. This would be of purely cosmetic interest were it not for the fact that osteoporosis is often accompanied by postural strain and mechanical damage.

This is a contributory cause of back pain in many elderly people. In North America, it is estimated that one out of every four women over the age of 60 years suffers from osteoporosis, an incidence which grows higher still once they have reached their allotted three-score-and-ten. By 90 years of age, every other woman can expect to have X-ray evidence of vertebral fracture, associated with osteoporosis. One defence against these degenerative changes is to eat plenty of calcium and Vitamin D. At present, about 30 per cent of adult women, and a similar proportion of men over the age of 70 years are believed to be suffering from calcium deficiency. This risk is particularly great in people who:
a) are on low-cholesterol diets (since dairy products are our major source of calcium);

b) drink to excess (because alcohol retards the absorption of calcium from the gut);

c) are heavy coffee-drinkers (a recent study at Washington State University reveals that drinking as little as three cups of coffee a day can impair calcium status);

d) eliminate bread from their diet in an attempt to lose weight (since bread is another rich source of calcium);

e) live in soft water areas (since these waters have a low mineral content).

There are probably several reasons for the prevalence of calcium deficiency today. For one thing, we lead less active lives than our forebears, which means that we have to restrict our overall intake of food to avoid becoming obese. This entails a reduction in our total consumption of calcium, which, although widely distributed in the foods we eat, is generally present in only small quantities. Some nutritionalists point out that we have increased our risk of running short of calcium by giving up our primitive forebears' habit of gnawing bones and swallowing the easily masticated bones of small fish. Anyone who eats the bones as well as the flesh of a 3 oz (90 g) serving of sardines for instance, will get a massive 370 mg shot of calcium, which is nearly half the recommended daily dose.

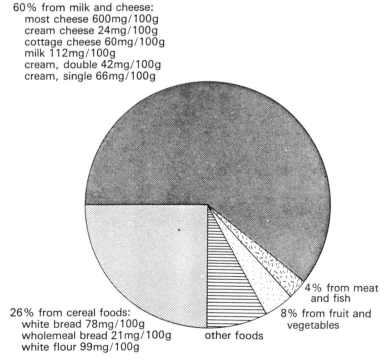

60% from milk and cheese:
   most cheese 600mg/100g
   cream cheese 24mg/100g
   cottage cheese 60mg/100g
   milk 112mg/100g
   cream, double 42mg/100g
   cream, single 66mg/100g

4% from meat and fish

8% from fruit and vegetables

26% from cereal foods:
   white bread 78mg/100g
   wholemeal bread 21mg/100g
   white flour 99mg/100g

other foods

Figure 28 Dietary sources of calcium.

The pie-chart (Figure 28) shows the major sources of calcium. If you want to maintain your skeletal health, eat plenty of dairy foods: milk, which supplies about 300 mg of calcium per glass, and cheese, which contains about 200 mg per 1 oz (30 g) helping. If you are anxious to cut down your intake of Calories or animal fats, drink skimmed milk rather than whole milk, for this has far less cholesterol, only half as many Calories and yet almost exactly the same content of calcium. Try also to eat three or four slices of wholemeal bread a day (50 mg of calcium per slice), together with plenty of green vegetables. (If you use the cooking water to make gravies, stocks and soups, you will make full use of the minerals which are leached out during the boiling process and which would otherwise be discarded down the drain.)

The third essential ingredient in a rational anti-lumbago diet is Vitamin D, which is vital for the uptake and conversion of calcium and phosphorus into healthy bone tissue. In children, a deficiency of Vitamin D leads to rickets, a disease characterised by softening and deformity of the growing bones. In adults, a lack of Vitamin D can cause a similar weakening of the bone structure, which at this time of life is generally called osteomalacia. It can also contribute to the development of osteo-porosis. Dairy foods, such as eggs, milk, butter and cheese, provide the major dietary sources of Vitamin D. Other rich sources are fish oils and fatty fish, such as mackerel and herrings. But there is a more important source of Vitamin D, which has nothing to do with the food we eat. Vitamin D has been called the sunshine vitamin because it can be created within the skin by the action of ultraviolet light on a naturally occurring vitamin precursor called ergosterol. This is almost certainly the major source of Vitamin D. The youngsters most prone to suffer rickets are those brought up in sun-starved cities. In the same way, the incidence of osteomalacia is high in nuns wearing habits which shield their skins from the sun's rays and in factory workers engaged in night shifts.

Recent research has shown that the blood levels of Vitamin D show a seasonal variation, being at their highest in the summer and at their lowest in the dark, winter months. This is linked to exposure to sunlight, but bears no relationship to the vitamin content of the diet. In the same way, it has been found that men deprived of sunlight, in submarines or during Arctic winters, show a low level of Vitamin D in their blood, even when their dietary intake of Vitamin D is high. This evidence suggests that sunbathing is the single most important factor in determining Vitamin D status.

This was confirmed by work carried out by the British Medical Research Council. They studied a group of over 100 pensioners attend-ing a hospital in Harrow, Middlesex, and found that, while many were existing on diets deficient in Vitamin D, only those who rarely went out in the sun showed signs of poor bone texture. As the Council concluded: 'Too little attention has been given to the role of sunlight in osteomalacia'.

Tests have shown that the Vitamin D status of elderly people can be improved by giving them daily sun baths, whereas a nutritional study at Cambridge University has revealed that blood levels of Vitamin D are little changed by giving oral doses of Vitamin D, even at twice or four times the recommended daily level. From this, the researcher concluded that Vitamin D deficiency in the elderly was 'a direct consequence of an indoor life style'. The answer to osteomalacia and senile fractures was to expose the body to the sun rather than to take Vitamin D supplements which he said were 'ineffective, unnatural and potentially dangerous'.

Unfortunately, in many temperate climates, it is often too cold to sit out in the open air in the Spring or Autumn, even on sunny days, owing to the chilling effect of the prevailing winds. Basking indoors in the sun's rays is no substitute, for conventional window-glass screens off most of the sun's precious ultraviolet rays. One exciting compromise has been discovered by a British firm, Travisglen Ltd of Swindon, who are marketing a range of solar conservatories, fitted with special glazing panels which transmit about 90 per cent of the sun's ultraviolet rays. Within these 'consolatries', it is possible to get bronzed in comfort even in the depth of winter. Tests in a Glasgow hospital show that only a trace of ultraviolet light penetrates the geriatric wards in January. If patients, or the inmates of old folks' homes, are placed in solar conservatories at this time, they would receive twenty-seven times the exposure of ultraviolet light. In March, the difference is greater still. As the days lengthen, the strength of the sun grows and yet it generally remains too cold to sit outdoors. Inside the hospital ward, very little ultraviolet light enters but, in the solar conservatory, the irradiation level leaps by well over a thousand times.

No doubt many geriatric wards and retirement homes in the future will be equipped with solar conservatories, for this single measure would go a long way to preventing osteoporosis and fractures of the hip, which currently occupy one in ten of all orthopaedic beds in the UK. A sensible anti-lumbago diet should therefore contain not only an adequate allowance of calcium and Vitamins C and D, but also plenty of sunshine.

VERDICT   People of all ages should ensure that they obtain an adequate supply of those nutrients which are necessary for the formation of sturdy bones and healthy joint tissues. This is particularly important for the over–60s who are most prone to degenerative joint diseases and also most likely to be on deficient diets. Younger adults tend to have a different dietary problem. Their troubles normally stem from overnutrition rather than undernutrition. They overeat, become obese and so subject their backs to unnecessary postural strain. For them an anti-lumbago diet is primarily one which is nourishing but Calorie-controlled.

26 Back-Up Treatment

The vast majority of acute back injuries get better spontaneously in 7–10 days, without the help of doctors or osteopaths, and a high proportion of chronic back problems can be relieved by the simple, self-help measures which have just been described. When pain persists despite these means, expert assistance should be sought. Nobody should resign themselves to a life of stubborn stoicism without a fight, or seek to make a virtue of martyrdom, for most cases of persistent spinal pain can be overcome with specialist help. The range of available treatment is wide and includes:

☆ *Injections* During recent years, just about every structure of the back has been the target of injections by local anaesthetics, anti-inflammatory agents, disc-dissolving enzymes and irritating chemicals designed to stimulate the formation of fibrous tissue. The results of these experiments have been sometimes good, sometimes useless and sometimes positively hazardous. The most successful injections have been those directed to specific painful muscle lumps (see p. 106).

Less success has been experienced with cortisone injections into the spinal canal, which were introduced to reduce the inflammation of nerves trapped by disc protrusions. Early results suggested this might prove to be a promising treatment of acute sciatica. In one trial, three-quarters of patients suffering from acute sciatica were improved or cured by these epidural injections. This gave reason for hope. Then it was found that exactly the same results were obtained by injecting an inert saline solution or by pricking the skin with the injection needle without actually entering the spinal canal. Whatever improvements occurred must have been due to the placebo effect or to the passage of time which normally brings about the resolution of acute sciatica.

False excitement was also aroused in the early 1960s by the introduction of injections designed to shrink the intervertebral discs. The substance used was chymopapain, an enzyme derived from the papaya fruit, which has been used for years to tenderize meat. Early tests on the spines of rabbits and dogs showed that intervetebral discs shrink when injected with chymopapain. This can even be demonstrated in the laboratory.

Drop a portion of human disc material into a test tube of chymopapain and it will dissolve within a few hours. These discoveries led to hopes that discs could be shrunk chemically rather than removed surgically, which would be much more acceptable to the patient and which would reduce by half the length of time spent in hospital. In the first fever of excitement, tens of thousands of people underwent chemonucleolysis, the term coined to describe the new technique. Early reports were encouraging. Then it was discovered that the procedure was not as benign as was at first thought. Some patients were allergic to chymopapain, others suffered a permanent scarring or painful inflammation of the disc after the injections (discitis). In one American survey, it was found that 1.7 per cent of people receiving a chymopapain injection suffer a marked allergic reaction from which one in 700 die. There are also doubts about the long-term effectiveness of chemonucleolysis. Injections of chymopapain undoubtedly shrink disc material but not always where this is required and, after a few months, scar tissue is formed around the injection site which may cause more trouble than the original disc protrusion. This may explain the method's high failure rate, which, according to a recent survey, runs as high as 50 per cent.

A number of doctors also use injections to strengthen spinal ligaments which are weak or overstretched. The substance used is frequently ethanolamine oleate, the chemical used to close distended varicose veins. The effect is to set up an irritation which stimulates the formation of new fibrous tissue. This reaction can be used to seal bulging veins or equally well to buttress weak ligaments.

☆ *Surgery* When back pain or sciatica persists, and there is clear X-ray evidence of a disc protrusion pressing on a spinal nerve, the decision may be taken to perform a spinal decompression operation. This involves removing part or all of the damaged disc (partial or complete laminectomy) and sometimes also includes the fixation of adjacent vertebrae to give the spine added stability (spinal fusion). The operation is done under a general anaesthetic and, providing there are no complications, the patient is usually free to walk within a few days and able to return to light work tasks within 4 to 6 weeks. Sometimes the results of surgery are excellent. Joss Naylor, Britain's champion fell-runner, has had several operations on his back, yet he has been able to set up records for speed ascents of mountain peaks of 2,000 ft (600 m) or more in the course of a single day, an incredible feat for a man with a bad back who at one time couldn't walk more than 50 yards! Unfortunately results like this cannot be guaranteed. After back surgery, many patients suffer recurrent pain in their back or leg, numbness, weakness or pain when standing, lifting and stooping. One teaching hospital in Norfolk, Virginia, carried out a 5-year study to determine the outcome of back surgery. The results tallied with previous surveys, revealing that approximately 64 per cent of patients responded satisfactorily, while in 24 per cent the response was poor and 12 per cent were classed as 'frank failures'. Slightly more than one in four developed recurrent back problems and approximately one in seven needed a second operation.

Spine operations should be performed only when all else fails, and pain persists for more than 6 months. People frequently criticise the long queues for back surgery at British hospitals, but the prolonged waits serve one very important function – they give people time to get better on their own accord without medical intervention. According to one estimate, two-thirds of Britons due for spinal surgery recover spontaneously while waiting for a hospital bed to become available!

☆ *Manipulation* Many people consider this to be the treatment of choice for back problems whether it is given by doctor, osteopath, chiropractor, physiotherapist or bonesetter. It is particularly valuable in chronic cases where pain is associated with stiffness of the muscles, ligaments and joints and can occasionally be of dramatic benefit in cases of acute back pain. These are the spectacular instances when patients struggle into an osteopath's consulting room doubled up with pain and bound out 15 minutes later, ramrod straight and free of pain. These miracles are the bane of my life, even though they may be excellent practice-builders, for every back-pain sufferer who enjoys a wave-of-the-wand cure recommends another twenty victims who are programmed to expect equally rapid results. Generally the response to manipulative treatment is much slower, certainly in cases of backache which have persisted unchanged for several years or which are accompanied by sciatic pain. In cases of uncomplicated backache, patients can generally be restored to health within about a fortnight. This was proved in a Danish study carried out at the Department of Rheumatology, Odense University Hospital. In this trial, a comparison was made of the effectiveness of manipulation and short-wave radiation in the relief of back pain. The results showed that 92 per cent of patients treated by manipulation were out of pain, free of all disablement and able to work within 14 days, compared with only 25 per cent of those who received short-wave therapy.

The risks of manipulation appear to be small, even in untutored hands, for the patient who is inadvisably or maladroitly manipulated generally suffers no more than an aggravation of their pain, from which they soon recover. The chief advantage of going to a skilled, trained manipulator is that they have the expertise to know *when* and *where* to manipulate as well as *how* to manipulate. Their training in diagnosis enables them to get results where others fail and also allows them to pick out those cases that are not suitable for manipulation.

☆ *Acupuncture* The use of this specialised method of treatment has already been considered in this book. Visiting a professional acupuncturist may be more effective than using the self-help measures outlined on page 119, but at present there is no evidence that this is so.

☆ *Drugs* The main line of treatment offered by family doctors is bed rest and pills. The drugs fall into three main categories: painkillers, muscle relaxants and anti-inflammatory agents. All these medicaments are palliative rather than curative, helping to relieve symptoms rather than eradicate root causes. The commonest anti-inflammatory agents are indomethacin (Indocid), phenylbutazone (Butazolidin), ibuprofen (Brufen), naproxen (Naprosyn), ketoprofen (Orudis), diclofenac (Voltarol) and piroxicam (Feldene). These are useful when there is evidence of inflammatory joint disease or irritation of the spinal nerves. Their greatest drawback is that they often give rise to an unacceptable level of nausea and indigestion, even when they are taken with food as instructed.

The favoured painkillers, among a vast range, are paracetamol, dextropropoxyphene (Distalgesic) and dihydrocodein (DF 118). Even these may not be strong enough to deaden the pain of severe lumbago or sciatica and may prove little advance on the simple remedies outlined on page 115. The common muscle relaxants are diazepam (Valium), meprobamate (Equanil) and mephenesin (Myanesin). These are designed to relax painful muscle spasm but in practice are disappointing and often no more effective than a hot bath. Sleeping pills also have their use in providing an untroubled night's rest.

☆ *Transcutaneous nerve stimulation* Three hundred years before the birth of Christ, the Greeks developed a treatment for lumbago which has only recently been resurrected in slightly more scientific form. Aristotle told how pain could be relieved by bringing a stingray in contact with the skin. A few decades later the Romans were getting the same analgesic effect by using electric eels and torpedo rays. In the eighteenth century, Benjamin Franklin introduced electrical shock machines into hospital practice and, 100 years later, Sarlandière, a French physician, developed an electro-acupuncture device for easing the pain of rheumatic disease. Now we use a box connected by electrodes to the skin which transmits tiny electric shocks. This is known as transcutaneous nerve stimulation or TNS. This acts in the same way as acupuncture, either by jamming the reception of pain stimuli or by increasing the output of the body's own anodynes, known as endorphins (see page 118). The results of using this device vary enormously. In one trial, TNS proved no more effective than a dummy device which was attached to the patient's body but which emitted no electrical impulses. In other instances, patients have claimed to gain relief by wearing a TNS stimulator and giving themselves a burst of tiny shocks whenever they needed to ease their pain.

☆ *Postural correction*   Where chronic back pain is associated with obvious postural faults, and is aggravated by excessive standing and stooping, it can often be relieved by a course of postural re-education given by either a physiotherapist or a teacher trained in the Alexander method.

☆ *Corsets*   Every year in the UK, about half a million spinal corsets are dispensed. For some strange reason, the prescription rate is twice as high in England as Scotland, possibly because the Sassenachs are a less stoical race! They should only be worn for a brief while in the early stages of an attack of acute lumbago, for the reasons outlined on page 99. They can also ease the postural strain of an exaggerated lumbar curve where patients are too old or too lazy to overcome the fault by correcting their obesity and carrying out exercises to strengthen their abdominal muscles and stretch out their contracted lumbar muscles.

27 Bangles, Belts And Bees

It would take an entire book, many times larger than this, to provide a complete compendium of country cures for lumbago and sciatica. Here is my personal choice of seventeen of the most helpful items of folk wisdom. (It had to be a prime number or the selection would have been stripped of its magic potency!)

1. COPPER BRACELETS

When the early Dutch settlers arrived in Rhodesia, they found that the indigenous population rarely suffered from rheumatic ailments. The natives attributed this immunity to their habit of wearing copper ornaments. This has now become a popular folk cure for rheumatism. Prince Philip sports one to improve the arthritis in his wrist; so too does the Marquess of Bath, who is reported to have been free of rheumatism since wearing the copper bangles which he now sells at the gift shop on his Longleat estate at the rate of 100 per week.

The use of a copper bangle is based on the ancient idea that rheumatism is due to the accumulation of impurities within the body. African witch-doctors traditionally suck the flesh of their patients to extract this noxious material, which they then spit out on the ground with a dramatic flourish. Elisha Perkins, one of the USA's earliest and most notorious medical quacks, used a similar principle to cure lumbago and sciatica. He developed a 'tractor', a device consisting of two metal rods which was said to extract sickness and pain when rubbed up and down a sufferer's back. In the UK, generations of country folk have endeavoured to achieve the same effect by wearing close to the skin a piece of copper or a portion of cut potato. When these charms turn black, as they inevitably will from exposure to the oxygen in the air, it is taken as a sure sign that the rheumatic impurities are being leached from the body.

Today this theory is rarely advanced. In this scientific age of silicon chips, it is considered more credible to suggest that wearing a copper bracelet sets up a protective galvanic field around the body. At present, it is estimated that 5 million Americans wear copper bangles and ornaments to ease their rheumatic aches and pains. But is there any evidence that the remedy works?

In Australia, medical researcher Professor W.R. Walker of the University of Newcastle has studied the subject and found that the weight of a copper bracelet worn to alleviate rheumatism decreases by an average of 40 mg a month. He believes that this steady attrition is possibly due to the dissolution of particles of copper in human sweat and its subsequent combination with the natural amino acids secreted by the skin's sebaceous glands. If this is true, it is just possible that some of the copper may be absorbed into the body, where it may exert an anti-inflammatory effect, just as gold salts do when given in the treatment of rheumatoid arthritis.

It seems more likely that the success and current popularity of the copper bracelet remedy rests on the fact that nine out of ten episodes of backache clear up spontaneously, with or without treatment, in about 10 days. No doubt, if a copper bracelet is worn during this time, it will get the kudos for the healing rather than Dame Nature.

2. MUSTARD PACK

This was a favourite remedy of Dr W.S.C. Copeman who, for many years, was consultant to the British Red Cross Clinic for Rheumatism at Peto Place, London. His instructions are as follows: dissolve 1 tablespoonful (20 g) of mustard in 1 pint (0.5 litres) of boiling water. Place into this mixture a towel folded to a size convenient to cover the lower back. When the towel is thoroughly soaked, squeeze it lightly to remove the excess liquid and then place it directly on the back as hot as can be borne. As mustard is a powerful counter-irritant it should not be left in contact with the skin for longer than 10 minutes, otherwise blistering can occur. Carry out this procedure once a day until the pain disappears.

3. MUSSEL DEVELOPMENT

A recent addition to the long line of country remedies for rheumatism is the New Zealand green-lipped mussel, better known to its friends as *Perna canaliculus*. This developed quite a reputation in its native country before its commercial potential was spotted and it was packaged for worldwide exploitation. For some reason, man has a great belief in the curative powers of slimy marine creatures. Oysters are a favourite aphrodisiac. Jellied eels are the native Londoner's pick-me-up and Hawaiian islanders swear by the therapeutic properties of a certain sea worm. (Tests show that extracts of the tentacles of this worm have an anti-carcinogenic effect on laboratory mice, although it has proved impossible to isolate the active ingredient.)

When patients first began to bring me glowing reports of the benefits they had derived from taking extracts of green-lipped mussel, I was inclined to suspect the placebo effect, particularly when they told me that the mussel could only be obtained from one particular New Zealand beach. Now I am not so sure. One thing in particular altered my evaluation of this exotic cure and that was a controlled trial carried out at the Victoria Infirmary, Glasgow. In this test, patients suffering from arthritis were given either an extract of *Perna canaliculus* or an identical-tasting dummy substance. Neither the patients nor the doctors conducting the experiment knew at any time which particular substance was being given. When the results were analysed at the end of 6 months' treatment, the researchers concluded that the new preparation 'reduces the amount of pain and stiffness, improves the patient's ability to cope with life and apparently enhances general health'. They found that 76 per cent of patients suffering from rheumatoid arthritis benefited from the remedy and about 45 per cent of those suffering from osteo-arthritis. From this, it appears that the anti-inflammatory properties of the green-lipped mussel are just as strong as those of the gold salts often used by rheumatologists, with a much lower risk of adverse side effects.

Back sufferers who find it difficult to sleep at night, and who suffer considerable stiffness and discomfort when they wake in the morning, may derive benefit from taking one 350 mg capsule of mussel extract before retiring to bed. The only common side effects are nausea, indigestion and flatulence. These are mild discomforts experienced by about one in seven takers. The capsules can be obtained without prescription from most pharmacies and health-food stores.

4. THE LECTERN DESK

In Victorian times it was customary for shipping clerks, teachers and tally-men to stand up to work. They spent hours every day pouring over papers arranged on high desks with sloping tops. This meant that their backs were far less stooped than those of their counterparts today, who normally work in a slumped, sedentary position. This position gave the Victorian scribes more freedom of movement and enabled them to shift their weight from side to side and so vary the strain on the spinal muscles and ligaments. Ernest Hemingway, a regular victim of back pains, found it more comfortable to work standing up.

Some businessmen today have reverted to a similar working arrangement, which they find far kinder to their backs. This is particularly true in New York where the stand-up desk has become something of a status symbol among the city's top executives. Roger Birk, chairman of stockbrokers Merrill, Lynch and Co., acquired his walnut lectern desk 14 years ago, in an attempt to ease crippling backaches brought on by long spells of sitting. With the aid of the desk, which he uses for all his routine work, Birk has overcome his pain. 'I find it pleasant and more practical than normal desks and even tension easing', he reports. George Shinn, chairman of First Boston Corporation, a leading merchant bank, is another executive who prefers to be on top of his work. He had his stand-up desk specially constructed for him from sketches he drew of an ancient teacher's lectern. He too finds the upright position more comfortable for work. At the Xerox Corporation, chairman C. Peter McColough has used a stand-up desk for over 20 years and persistent back pain has recently forced his President, David T. Kearns, to follow suit.

Unfortunately stand-up desks are not readily attainable but they could be easily constructed for anyone who wants to try this simple way of relieving the postural strain of their work.

5. THE MAYO COCKTAIL

Numerous studies of patients suffering from backache and arthritis have shown that they eat practically the same diet as everyone else. A few have signs of vitamin deficiency but then so has a large proportion of the general population and there is no evidence that taking vitamin supplements, even in megadoses, has a beneficial effect on the course of any of the rheumatic diseases. Despite this, many people believe that large helpings of fruit can help to cure arthritic pain. Adelle Davis, the famous American nutritionalist, held this opinion. She thought that a deficiency of Vitamin C, by causing an increased fragility of the blood-vessel walls, led to painful bleeding into the joints when they were subjected to minor injury. 'These tiny haemorrhages', she wrote, 'occur first in the intestinal walls, the bone marrow, and joints, sometimes causing pain spoken of as "rheumatism".'

Despite the lack of supporting clinical evidence, there may be some validity in this argument. In any case, most people would benefit by eating more fruit and fresh green vegetables. Some may even like to try the Mayo Cocktail, a popular remedy for rheumatism which is said to have originated from the famous Mayo Clinic in Rochester, Minnesota. The ingredients are: three lemons, three oranges, three grapefruits and 2 oz (60 g) each of Epsom salts and cream of tartar. To make up the cocktail, express the juice from the fruits and thoroughly liquidise the skins, pulp and pips. Mix together with 2 pints (1 litre) of boiling water and leave to stand overnight. The next day strain the mixture slowly through a muslin cloth, then add the Epsom salts and cream of tartar and a further pint (0.5 litres) of boiling water. Store in the refrigerator until required. Shake well before use and take one full wine glass every morning before breakfast for at least 6 months.

6. NO SMOKE WITHOUT FIRE

Back pain is often aggravated by coughing, sneezing or going to the toilet and straining to pass a motion. In severe cases of sciatica, sometimes even laughing is no joke. This relationship is easily explained. Every time we strain, the diaphragm descends. This puts pressure on the blood inside the intra-abdominal veins, including those which travel in close association with the spinal nerves. This makes the veins dilate and apply pressure against the nerves, particularly where they leave the spine. If the nerve fibres at this site are already pinched or inflamed, every cough produces an additional stab of pain. This is why sciatic victims often grab their backs before they sneeze and bend their knees to take the tension off the roots of the sciatic nerve.

Repeated coughing is liable to aggravate any back complaint involving nerve-root compression. This no doubt is why smokers have an above-average risk of suffering back pains. This link was confirmed in an investigation of over 500 adults in the New Haven and Hartford areas of Connecticut. This showed that there were three main factors which showed a statistically significant tendency to increase the risk of suffering severe back problems. These were car driving, working in jobs involving heavy twisting and lifting, and smoking ten or more cigarettes a day. Other activities which are often thought to provoke spinal troubles, such as wearing high-heeled shoes, jogging or bearing a number of children, were not found to be associated with an increased liability to spinal injuries.

Research carried out by Professor Malcolm Jayson and his colleagues at the Rheumatic Disease Centre, Manchester, shows that victims of back pain often show abnormalities in their handling of fibrin, the sub-stance which is formed in the early stages of wound repair. Trials show that this repair tissue is more easily dispersed in healthy subjects than in people subject to severe back pain, in whom it possibly persists around the site of a wound, giving rise to inflammation, scarring and adhesion formation. This discovery may help to explain the smoker's predisposi-tion to back pain, for previous studies have shown that smokers suffer impaired fibrinolysis, the enzyme system responsible for the breakdown of fibrin clots.

It would appear from this evidence that back pain must now be added to the long list of diseases caused by cigarette smoking. Certainly anyone who suffers chronic back pain is well advised to quit cigarettes or, at the very least, to switch to smoking a pipe which carries a reduced risk of damaging the back.

7. COUNTING ON SHEEP

An ancient remedy for insomnia is to lie back and take an imaginary count of sheep jumping a fence. Sheep play an even more tangible role in a recently discovered cure for nocturnal rheumatism. Many people with aches and pains in their limbs and back claim that they get a better night's sleep when they are lying on a lambswool underblanket.

The idea stems from the chance discovery by a 72-year-old New Zealander, whose arthritis was making it increasingly difficult for him to fall asleep. One night the pain was so severe that, in desperation, he quit his bed and lay on the floor wrapped in a lambswool rug. Within minutes he had fallen asleep and, when he awoke in the morning, he realized that he had enjoyed the best night's rest for months. So, for the next three nights, he repeated the experiment, with similar results. Then he tried using the rug as an underblanket on his bed. This added to his comfort.

The news quickly spread and, in a country more densely populated with sheep than people, he soon had many followers who were equally convinced of the value of sleeping on a bed of fleece. The idea was then tested by one of the country's leading universities. The report, published in the *Medical Journal of Australia* in 1984, disclosed that 90 per cent of a group of over 700 sufferers from chronic rheumatism and arthritis derived benefit from sleeping on a lambswool underlay.

Why is this? Possibly the fleece, which traps a large volume of air within its mesh of fibres, provides a warm and resilient air cushion which supports the body and takes excessive pressure away from painful spots around the pelvis, shoulders and knees. As the remedy is relatively cheap, totally harmless, durable and pleasant to use, it might be worth a try by anyone suffering from chronic backache, particularly when the pain makes sleeping difficult.

An alternative is to sleep on underlays filled with pure cotton, such as have been used in China for nearly 3,000 years. These too provide a resilient support with good insulating properties and, in one trial, were shown to give relief to rheumatism or back pain in 48 per cent of cases.

8. BELOW THE BELT

Dr Gustave Jaeger, founder of the famous chain of shops which bears his name, was a pioneer of the dress-reform movement which flourished towards the end of the nineteenth century. He believed that good health could be maintained only by encasing the body in clothes made exclusively of wool. This was essential, he said, to keep the body warm, to facilitate the loss of waste products through perspiration and to ensure the equal distribution of blood throughout the body. (He believed that men walked about with pot bellies and spindly legs because the clothes they wore overheated their stomachs but kept their legs cold!) He advised his patients and dedicated followers, who came to be known as 'woolleners', to wear sanitary woollen shirts, sanitary woollen body belts and sanitary woollen combinations specially designed to keep out draughts. Nowadays we generally wear much lighter underclothing but many sufferers from backache still wear woollen body belts to keep out the cold winter winds. This is a protective measure of great antiquity, first mentioned in the Old Testament (Proverbs 31: 21), where it is reported that the perfect Jewish wife 'fears not snow for her household for they all wear scarlet wool'.

Earlier in this book, it was pointed out that muscular back pains can sometimes result from localised chilling of the back, especially when the muscles are being held in a state of sustained contraction (page 102). One way of preventing this is by protecting the back with a layer of clothing with a high insulation value. Normally, our clothes hold somewhere in the region of 50 pints (36 litres) of air. The more air we trap around the body, the better the insulation. For this reason, two layers of thin under-clothing give better protection than one thicker layer, particularly if they have an open weave. Natural fibres are generally better insulators than the denser synthetic fibres because they trap more air around the body. This is particularly true of wool, which, unlike cotton, has a natural resilience that makes it resist compression.

For these reasons, a number of doctors today still recommend woollen body belts as a protection against lumbago, particularly for people who work out of doors in draughty situations.

9. SIGH OF RELIEF

Rarely a day goes by without my getting a 'phone call from a patient who is in desperate need of help. They have made an awkward movement and now they are locked with pain. They would dearly love to come for treatment but have only just managed to struggle to the telephone. Making the journey to my consulting rooms is out of the question. What should they do?

Every osteopath has his or her own pet answer to this particular plea. My advice varies according to the circumstances of the case. Often I resort to a ruse used by my late friend and colleague Edward Hall, a dedicated osteopath who spent his entire life studying and teaching the practice and principles of osteopathy. He advised his immobilised patients to spend a few minutes breathing as slowly and deeply as possible. This simple exercise may seem to have little connection with the back but it can often unlock painful spinal muscle spasm enough to get the victims out of their muscular vice and allow them to take their first faltering steps.

It works in two main ways. In the first place, deep breathing is relaxing, particularly when emphasis is placed on the phase of expiration. Breathe out slowly and deeply, as if you were giving a sigh of relief, and muscle tension is automatically reduced. Deep breathing also hastens the return of blood from the abdomen to the heart. When the diaphragm descends,

143

it puts pressure on the veins within the abdomen and also on those surrounding the emerging spinal nerves. Doing this suddenly, with a cough or a sneeze, can be agonising for anyone with a pinched spinal nerve, but doing it gradually and rhythmically can help to relieve the hydrostatic pressure on the trapped nerve root by pumping blood away from the abdominal cavity back to the heart.

10. THE NAPOLEONIC APPROACH

Few people appreciate the potency of the human imagination. Tell a man under hypnosis that he is locked in a refrigeration van and he will not only shiver and feel cold but will also develop goose pimples and show a drop in skin temperature. Touch him with a stick and say that it is a red hot poker and he will wince with pain and possibly also develop a red weal and maybe even a blister. Such is the power of the subconscious mind, a largely untapped human resource. 'Imagination', said Napoleon, 'rules the world'.

Earlier this century, Emil Coué, the father of autosuggestion, demonstrated how the powers of the subconscious mind could be harnessed to heal the sick. Many doctors today are rediscovering the value of this approach, particularly in the relief of pain and in the fight against cancer. Here are some useful ways of easing back pain, derived from techniques employed at pain relief centres such as the Pain and Health Rehabilitation Center, in La Crosse, Wisconsin, and the Cancer Counselling and Research Center in Fort Worth, Texas:

To harness your body's innate healing powers, imagine your back becoming warm from an influx of blood. Then visualize the blood cells tackling their reparative work. In your mind's eye, watch the fibroblasts healing the damaged fibrous tissues and sense the growing comfort as the endorphins, the body's natural opiates, go about their work of pain relief.

Try to distance yourself from the pain and tension in your back. Imagine that your spine belongs to somebody else and that you are a healer standing close by. Now reach down and begin to massage the stranger's back slowly and gently. Give them as much support and relief as you can. Then, when the pain has eased, take possession of your body again.

Visualize your pain as being transmitted along a network of telephone wires from your brain to your back. Then take a pair of pincers and carefully cut the connections strand by strand. As you do so, feel the drop in pain intensity as you cut each individual wire. Do this exercise slowly and methodically, pacing yourself so that the last sensation of discomfort disappears as you sever the final thread.

11. HERBAL TEA

Feverfew is a daisy-like plant with a strong scent. It stands about 2 ft (60 cm) tall and grows like a weed in favourable soil. Its stems are straggly and its florets undistinguished and, because of its lack of elegance, it has been eliminated from the herbaceous borders of many country gardens, where pride of place is given to the more dramatically colourful delphiniums, lupins, phlox and Canterbury bells. But the humble feverfew once claimed a place in every garden, not so much because of its beauty as for its medicinal properties and magic powers. It was generally planted close to the front door of a house to bring good luck, purify the air and protect the occupants from disease.

It gained its botanical name – *Tanacetum parthenium* or Parthenium marigold – because, according to an ancient Greek legend, it was used in miraculous fashion to save the life of a workman who had fallen from the Parthenon while it was being built. Its popular name, feverfew, arose because it was most commonly employed as a febrifuge, to lower the temperature in fevers. It was also used as an antidote for giddiness and menstrual pain, and recently it has gained a reputation as a remedy for migraine and rheumatic pain.

There may be some justification for these claims, for research workers at the Miles Laboratory in Buckinghamshire have discovered that feverfew has a very similar action to aspirin, exerting an anti-inflammatory effect on the body by inhibiting the formation of substances known as prostaglandins. Some people simply eat the fresh, raw leaves, the recommended dose being one large or three small leaves per day. As the leaves have a bitter taste, they are best eaten with a cheese or savoury spread sandwich. A more palatable way of taking the herb is as a tea, an infusion being made by pouring a cup of boiling water on a heaped teaspoonful (5 g) of dried leaves. In this case, the dose is one or two cups per day. Supplies of dried feverfew can be obtained from herbalists and health-food stores.

12. BELLADONNA BALM

Early in my student days, I met Dr Harrison Fryette, a distinguished American osteopath who had a refreshingly practical approach to the treatment of back pain. He was an astute clinician and skilled manipulator but was not too proud to make use of country cures. One of his favourite remedies was those old-fashioned belladonna plasters, which are still available at chemist shops. In his book *Principles of Osteopathic Technique*, he wrote, 'A good old belladonna porous plaster placed over the sacroiliac and sacrolumbar area often gives a good deal of comfort'.

Belladonna has an ancient history. It is a medicinal herbal extract obtained from the root, leaves or berries of the deadly nightshade plant.

Rabbits, sheep and goats appear to be able to eat the herb with impunity and there is one report of a horse who suffered no ill effects after swallowing 8 lb (3.6 kg) of deadly nightshade. Children, on the other hand, can be killed by eating as few as two or three berries. This was the poison that Macbeth's troops are said to have used to kill an army of invading Danes.

The active ingredient of belladonna is atropine, a drug which has a profound effect on the autonomic nervous system. Its main medicinal use today is in the form of eyedrops, which dilate the pupils and facilitate the examination of the inside of the eye. The ladies of fashion in ancient Italy were aware of this effect and took minute doses of the deadly night-shade berry to widen their pupils and increase their sexual allure. This is how the herb gots its name belladonna, meaning 'beautiful lady'.

When applied externally, belladonna lessens irritability and pain. At one time, when nursing mothers developed mastitis, their painfully distended breasts were enveloped in belladonna plasters. Now the specially made porous plasters are used almost exclusively in the treat-ment of acute lumbago when they give both comfort and support. Because of their toxic properties they should never be applied over broken skin.

13. A STINGING SOLUTION

It is claimed that bee-keepers rarely succumb to lumbago or arthritis. Many members of the Bad Back Club also swear that they have been helped by bee-sting therapy. The late actor Jack Warner took this cure for his arthritis and reported: 'It certainly seems to work, once the pain of the sting goes'.

At one time, it was thought that bee stings provided a form of counter-irritation. Tests showed that the venom contained formic acid, a sub-stance which is highly irritating when injected under the skin. This chemical is also found in ant-stings and nettle-stings, which is why country folk in the UK were once advised to ease their aching joints by rolling naked in a bed of stinging nettles, and why natives of Siberia once treated their painful backs by rubbing them with a formic-acid poultice made from ants' nests. This was a highly effective treatment according to eye-witness Paul Kourennoff, whose family have been practitioners of country medicine for seven generations, and who says: 'I witnessed several complete cures involving people who were paralysed by crippling arthritis'.

More recent research reveals that the effectiveness of bee-sting therapy cannot be explained simply on the basis of its counter-irritant action. Tests show that the venom has a direct anti-inflammatory effect. Research workers at the Ohio University College of Osteopathic Medicine introduced killed bacteria into the foot pads of rats. This set up an inflammation which made the tissues swell but it was discovered that the degree of swelling was 30 per cent less when rats were given a protective shot of bee venom. No such change occurred when the rats were injected with an inert saline solution.

Further investigations succeeded in isolating one of the active anti-inflammatory constituents of bee venom, a substance called Peptide 401. Unfortunately, animal experiments revealed that this chemical provoked too many side effects to make it a useful medicinal drug. Subsequent research at University College, London, unearthed another fraction of bee venom which is as potent as Peptide 401, but much less toxic. This may prove to be an effective anti-rheumatic drug. Until it becomes available, back-sufferers will have to be content with old-fashioned bee-sting therapy, which is still available from specialist practitioners who are more often self taught then medically trained.

14. CHINESE KNUCKLING

Pain in the back can radiate from a number of sites, the most common being the muscles, ligaments, joints and spinal nerves. Occasionally discomfort seems to stem from the superficial tissues. People sometimes have flesh which is peculiarly sensitive to touch. Grip their flesh and they will wince. Subjectively, they will complain of feeling bruised, as if their spines have been trampled over by a regiment of soldiers in hob-nail boots. If you examine their skin, you will often find that it is puffy, lumpy and sometimes pitted with dimples. Doctors in the past used to refer to this condition as panniculitis. In cosmetic circles, it is more commonly known as *cellulite*, a French word which should not be confused with cellulitis, a medical term describing a generalised infection of the superficial tissues.

Many treatments have been advocated for overcoming panniculitis or *cellulite*, the most popular being a form of massage which draws the skin away from the deeper lying tissues. Beauticians today pinch the affected skin between their fingers and thumbs and then draw it away from the underlying muscles and bones with a series of lifting, rolling or kneading actions. The Egyptians covered the body with suction cups which they manipulated over painful areas of flesh like tiny vacuum cleaners. This ancient cupping therapy is still employed today by some alternative-medicine practitioners, especially in the treatment of lumbago, sciatica and fibrositis. The cups used nowadays are generally made of thick glass. These are heated by any convenient means so that the air inside them expands. The rim of the glass is then placed firmly against the painful portion of the back. As the air inside cools a partial vacuum is formed which draws the skin inwards inside the cup. This can have a beneficial

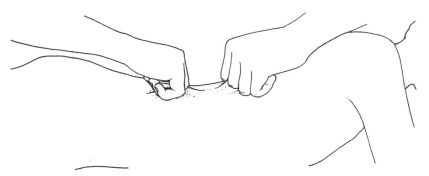

Figure 29 Chinese massage. Lifting up the skin between the knuckles.

effect in cases of chronic backache associated with superficial tenderness, possibly because it stretches the superficial connective tissues or because it improves the intimate circulation of the skin.

In China the same effect is obtained by gripping the skin between the crooked first and second fingers, as shown in Figure 29. This is as effective as cupping and much simpler to apply. What is more the technique requires equipment which is always to hand and carries no risk of painful burns. (I have seen patients with permanent, circular scars – looking like the glassmarks on a dining-room table – caused by intemperate cupping!)

15. THE JAPANESE BED-ROLL

High on the list of fiendish contraptions for straining the back are deckchairs, airport luggage carousels and foldaway beds for occasional guests. How often a weekend stay with family or friends is marred by a crippling bout of lumbago, brought on by spending a couple of nights on a camp bed, sun lounger, sofa or foldaway divan. These sleeping devices are cheap, easily stored and undoubtedly convenient for temporary use, but they can play havoc with sensitive spines. A more satisfactory solution is to make up a bed on the floor using a thin mattress which can be rolled away when not required. For centuries the Japanese have been sleeping in this way on *futons*, slim mattresses filled with layers of fleecy cotton. These are now generally obtainable. They provide comfortable support for the spine and are idea for overnight guests, or for regular use in one-room flats when they can be rolled up and tucked away in a cupboard during the day to create more space.

16. PELVIC PERCHES

Standing is never a comfortable posture for the back. Stand too long in this one position – in church, at a cocktail party or at the tail of a super-

148

market check-out queue – and the back muscles will quickly groan with fatigue and the spinal ligaments wince with postural strain. Primitive man had an easy answer to this problem: he rarely stood, preferring to while away his time squatting on his haunches or sitting cross-legged on the ground. Problems arose only with the march of civilisation when we adopted static pursuits. In our work we may stand for 6 or more hours a day teaching a class of children. In our play, we sometimes stand beside the rails of a racecourse and spend an entire afternoon following the horses. Even in our devotions we spend a long time on our feet. This was particularly true of the medieval monks, who would stand for hours during church services. Anyone engaged in these activities is prone to develop back pain and soon finds ways of taking the weight off the feet. Schoolteachers often sit on their desks in front of the class; regular racegoers will use a shooting stick, while medieval monks used their ingenuity to develop the misericord seat which enabled them to rest on their haunches while seeming to stay on their legs.

Senator Ted Kennedy crushed three vertebrae when he was involved in a plane crash in 1964. Since that time he has been liable to back pain, particularly when he stands at the end of a reception line shaking hands with a large number of voters; he alleviates the strain on his back by propping himself against a high, folding chair held by one of his Secret Service agents.

Any back sufferer who needs to stand for long periods should follow this example, using a shooting stick or folding, tripod chair to ease the prolonged postural strain on the back.

17.   CAUGHT IN THE ACT

More backs are injured in the bedroom than in the workshop, garden or kitchen. The standard consulting room query, 'How did you injure your back?', often evokes a sheepish grin or maidenly blush, which precedes the confession that it was strained while making love. The frequency of this embarrassing dilemma is not surprising. If you have a mechanical defect in your spine you are unlikely to disturb it walking down the street but you may upset it if you do something vigorous, like climb a five-barred gate or indulge in energetic sex. Since very many people have intercourse more often than they climb five-barred gates, this is the more common provoking factor. Sometimes a bad back is merely advanced as a useful excuse for avoiding sex. This is rarely justified, for most cases of chronic backache are *improved* rather than aggravated by the rhythmical movements of sexual intercourse. Horse-riding and pelvic-thrusting are useful exercises to mobilise a stiff lower back. (One young lady was questioned by the police when they spotted her standing by a bus stop one night doing her pelvic bumps!)

When back pain does limit sexual performance, it can be eased by adopting a more comfortable position. Most of the copulatory postures listed in the sex manuals are suitable only for contortionists and limbo dancers. The ones most appropriate for back-pain sufferers are the side-lying position and the conventional 'missionary' posture, with the patient taking the underneath berth so that the spine is supported by the bed or floor.

If this fails to give relief, an analgesic tablet should be taken half an hour before having sex.

28 The End In Sight

Confucius may have known precious little about bad backs but he had a very shrewd understanding of human nature. As a result he would have guessed, even 2,000 years ago, that many people would get to the end of this book feeling genuinely enthusiastic about what they had read. Somewhere in the preceding pages they would have discovered ways and means by which they could begin at last to master their chronic back problems. That realization would have brought them comfort and hope. But many of you reading this book are destined to get no further than this point. You will realize the rewards that are within your grasp but will not reach out and pluck them. This is the great tragedy of health education, that communication about the facts of illness does not cause automatic conversion to the ways of health. As Confucius said: 'The essence of knowledge is, having it, to apply it'.

This book provides the information necessary to help you overcome your back pains but it is powerless to assist if you are not prepared to pursue the practical guidance it gives. We often indulge in the game of wishful thinking. If only my back was strong enough, I'd dig the garden, learn judo or take up wind-surfing. If only I wasn't stiff in the morning when I struggle out of bed and try to put on my socks and shoes. If only I could stand at a cocktail party without getting a burning pain in the hollow of my back. All these dreams could come true, if we were only prepared to work to convert hopes into realities. This does not demand heroic effort or great self sacrifice. All that is needed is that you should take a tiny step forward on the way to cure every day.

A wise policy is to keep this book by your bedside so you can refresh your memory and strengthen your resolve by dipping into it from time to time. And once you have mastered your own problems please do your best to spread the good news to other sufferers. Join in the campaign to conquer the scourge of back pain. Don't let your friends suffer in silence. Point them to the way of cure. Lend them, or better still buy them, a copy of this book. Backache is the Cinderella disease of modern medical practice because it doesn't shorten life but it does destroy its quality. The Arabs express this in a most effective way. They say that health is the digit one, while love is zero, wealth zero, fame zero and success zero. Put the one of health before the others and you have all that anyone could desire. But without the one of health everything else remains nought. Overcome your back pain and you may not add years to your life, but you will add life to your years.

Glossary

Adhesion A band of fibrous tissue linking tissues that are normally unconnected. When formed within joints they can give rise to pain and limited movements.

Adolescent kyphosis An excessive rounding of the back occurring in youngsters, often caused by Scheuermann's disease (*q.v*).

Ankylosing spondylitis An inflammatory disease associated with progressive stiffening of the spine which is 5–10 times more common in men than in women.

Annulus fibrosus The outermost part of the discs between the vertebrae, made primarily of collagen fibres which are stronger than strands of steel of similar thickness.

Apophyseal joints The joints on either side of the vertebrae which give flexibility to the spine.

Arachnoiditis An inflammation of the connective tissues enveloping the spinal chord, most commonly encountered as a complication of myelography (*q.v.*).

Arthrodesis The fusion of a joint, an operative procedure sometimes applied to the spine to relieve pain and counteract instability.

Bamboo spine The X–ray appearance of the spine in ankylosing spondylitis (*q.v.*).

Bonesetters Untutored manipulators, generally found in rural communities.

Brucellosis (undulant fever) A bacterial infection, sometimes transmitted in unpasteurized milk, which can cause spinal disease and back pain.

Chemo-nucleolysis The use of injected chemicals to dissolve portions of the intervertebral discs.

Chiropractic The school of spinal manipulation developed by D.D.Palmer.

Chymopapain An enzyme derived from the papaya fruit, commonly used in the technique of chemo-nucleolysis (*q.v.*).

Coccygodynia (coccydynia) Pain experienced in the coccyx or tail bone, often resulting from a fall.

Collagen The fibrous protein which forms the basis of connective tissues such as ligaments, cartilage and skin.

Cortisone The steroid hormone produced by the outer layer (cortex) of the adrenal glands. Injection of cortisone derivatives are often used for their anti-inflammatory and pain-relieving properties.

Diathermy The generation of heat beneath the surface of the skin by a process of induction, short-wave electric currents being passed between two surface electrodes. Now thought to be no more effective than simpler forms of heat application, so less frequently used by physiotherapists than previously.

Discography The X–ray investigation of the intervertebral discs after the injection of a suitable contrast medium.

Electromyograph (EMG) A record of muscular activity based on a measurement of its electrical responses.

Endorphins The naturally-occurring pain-relieving substances released within the body in response to painful stimulation.

Epidural space The space inside the spinal column which lies between the bony vertebral canal and the tough sheath of connective tissue (dura) which envelops the spinal chord. This is the site for epidural injections.

Facet syndrome Painful symptoms arising from disorders of the apophyseal joints (q.v.).

Fascia lata The stout layer of connective tissue which runs from the pelvis to the knee. This is particularly well developed on the outer aspect of the thigh. Abnormal shortening of the fascia in this region is believed to be an occasional contributory cause of back pain and sciatica.

Femoral neuritis An involvement of the femoral nerve, similar to sciatica, but causing pain in the groin and front of the thigh.

Hemivertebrae A congenital anomaly in which one or more half vertebrae develop, invariably causing acute lateral curvature of the spine.

Herpes zoster (shingles) A virus disease, which can cause back pain and sciatica when it involves the lumbar nerves. This may not be accurately diagnosed until the characteristic skin rash appears, generally within about a week of the onset of the disease.

Ilio-lumbar ligaments The stout, triangular-shaped ligaments which run from the sides of the lowest lumbar vertebrae to the pelvis. They give lateral stability to the base of the spine and are a common site of strain.

Intermittent claudication A disorder characterised by painful cramps in the legs after walking a short distance. Caused by a restriction in the arterial blood supply, it is sometimes mistaken for sciatic pain.

Intervertebral foramina The apertures through which the roots of the spinal nerves leave the vertebral column. They are bordered in front by the intervertebral discs and behind by the arthrodial joints (q.v.), which makes them vulnerable to nerve compression.

'Kissing' spines The term used to describe the condition when the spinous processes, or knobs, at the back of the spine impinge on one another.

Kyphosis An exaggerated rounding, or forward curvature, of the spine.

Laminectomy An operation to remove the laminae or plates which form the roof of the spinal canal, generally performed to reduce pressure on the spinal cord and nerves.

Ligamenta flava The elastic ligaments which link the laminae (see **Laminectomy**) of adjacent vertebrae. When thickened they can cause pressure on the emerging spinal nerves.

'Locked back' syndrome A term sometimes used to describe episodes of sudden, painful fixation of the lower back, which can be caused by a variety of mechanical derangements.

Lordosis An increased hollowing of the back.

Lumbago A non-specific term used to describe pain in the lower, lumbar region of the spine whatever its cause.

Lumbar puncture An investigation in which a sample of fluid is taken from the spinal canal by inserting a long, hollow needle into the back. This test has little place in the routine examination of back problems and is less frequently used than previously owing to the discomfort and risks involved.

Maitland exercises A system of movements devised by Australian physiotherapist G.G. Maitland, frequently used by physiotherapists to loosen the spine.

Myelography The injection of a radio-opaque medium into the vertebral canal, to show up disc protrusions or tumours which would not otherwise be seen on X–rays.

Neural (vertebral) canal The tunnel at the back of the spine which houses the spinal chord.

Nipped synovial fringe A painful condition which arises when the lining membranes of the arthrodial joints (*q.v.*) are trapped between the opposing joint surfaces.

Nucleus pulposus The inner portion of each intervertebral disc contained within the annulus fibrosus (*q.v.*), which consists of incompressible, jelly-like material.

Osteoarthritis A form of degenerative joint disease, frequently found in the spine's arthrodial joints and often accompanied by spondylosis (*q.v.*).

Osteomalacia An abnormal softening of the bone caused by lack of the bone-strengthening materials calcium and phosphorus. Generally caused by a deficiency of Vitamin D.

Osteopathy A system of manipulation devised by Andrew Taylor Still, aimed at overcoming structural disorders in the body's locomotor apparatus.

Osteophytes Bony spurs found around joints affected by degenerative arthritis, commonly encountered around the vertebral bodies and arthrodial joints in spondylosis (*q.v.*).

Osteoporosis A weakening of the bone, commonly found in older women, associated with a deficiency of the protein framework, or matrix, of the bone tissue.

Paget's disease (osteitis deformans) A disease associated with painful enlargement and deformity of the bones, often affecting the lumbar spine.

Poker spine A term used to describe the rigid back found in ankylosing spondylitis. (*q.v.*).

Pott's disease Tuberculosis of the vertebrae, generally associated with marked, hump-backed deformity. Now rarely encountered.

Prolapsed intervertebral disc The condition, popularly but inaccurately, described as a 'slipped disc', in which the tough outer casing of the disc ruptures and, generally in company with bulging material from the nucleus pulposus (*q.v.*), presses on nearby pain-sensitive structures.

Reiter's disease A disease, generally associated with a non-specific inflammation of the urinary tracts (NSU), commonly affecting young men, which causes inflammation of the eye, a painful discharge from the penis and arthritis of the leg joints and sometimes those of the lower back.

Sacralization A condition in which the lowest lumbar vertebrae is fused to the sacrum and becomes a fixed part of the pelvis.

Sacro-iliac joints The joints between the sacrum and pelvis, frequently the site of strain in young people and pregnant women.

Sacrum The wedge-shaped bone, sandwiched between the two hip bones (ilia), on which the spine rests.

Scheuermann's disease A developmental disorder of the growing parts of the vertebral bodies, generally giving rise to an excessive rounding of the spine (see **Adolescent kyphosis**).

Schmorl's nodes A bulging of disc material into the vertebral bodies, commonly multiple and occurring in more than a third of spines.

Sciatica Pain of whatever cause radiating down the back of the leg along the distribution of the sciatic nerve.

Scoliosis A lateral or sideways curvature of the spine.

Senile kyphosis An increased rounding of the spine brought about by a loss of thickness of the spinal discs and often aggravated by a weakening of bone texture and consequent wedging of the vertebrae (see **Osteoporosis**).

Slipped disc see **Prolapsed intervertebral disc.**

Spina bifida A congenital deformity in which the spinal canal fails to close fully. In severe cases this may allow the nerve tissues to protrude through the spine.

Spinous processes The bony knobs at the back of the vertebrae which provide attachment for muscles, ligaments and fascia.

Spondylolisthesis A forward slipping of one or more vertebrae.

Spondylosis A degenerative process associated with a loss of resilience and thickness of the spinal discs, osteoarthritis of the arthrodial joints and the formation of osteophytes (*q.v.*) around the rim of the vertebral bodies.

Tomography A computer-aided scanning technique for obtaining sectional pictures of the body, known as computerized axial tomography or CAT.

Ultrasonography A method of measuring the diameter of the spinal canal by timing the echo produced by an ultrasonic beam.

Zygopophyseal joints An alternative name for arthrodial joints of the spine.

Index

158